AF477169

Study of Crude Drugs

Fifteenth Edition

Prof. Dr. M. A. IYENGAR
Former Faculty
Department of Pharmacognosy
Manipal College of Pharmaceutical Sciences
MANIPAL – 576 104
INDIA

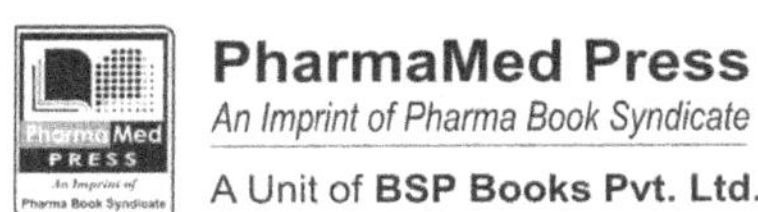

PharmaMed Press
An Imprint of Pharma Book Syndicate
A Unit of **BSP Books Pvt. Ltd.**

4-4-309/316, Giriraj Lane,
Sultan Bazar, Hyderabad - 500 095.

Study of Crude Drugs

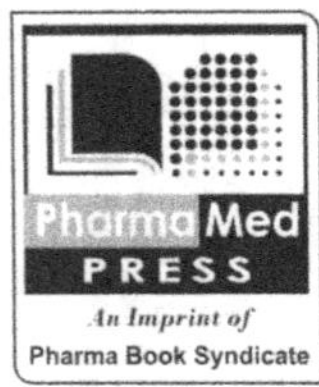

PharmaMed Press
An Imprint of Pharma Book Syndicate

A Unit of **BSP Books Pvt. Ltd.**

4-4-309/316, Giriraj Lane,
Sultan Bazar, Hyderabad - 500 095.

Pages	:	146 (13 + viii)
Photos	:	62
Line Diagrams	:	89

© 1981
2019 22nd Reprint

ISBN : 978-93-90211-13-5

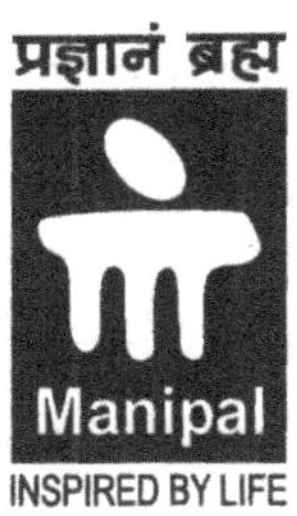

Dedicated to this place
MANIPAL

the halo that enshrines education
the sceptre that endows a healing touch
the light that guides the pride of tomorrow.

PREFACE   *First Edition*

It is gratifying to note the warm reception accorded to my books published hitherto and I take this opportunity to thank those numerous student friends and well-wishers whose encouragement stimulated me to continue in my venture. I hope this book too would receive the same warm treatment at their hands.

"Study of Crude Drugs" is a companion volume to the other books authored by me. The Pharmacy Council of India has thoroughly revised the syllabus. I on my part have tried to meet the requirements of the syllabus which however have not been defined properly. I have tried here to provide suitable material in the form of information and to present it in the way in which it may most easily be assimilated. One hundred and twentyfive drugs are dealt with in a set proforma. The information on chemistry is indicative rather than extensive. Everything in this book is intended to help the student to express himself correctly and fluently in Pharmacognosy and any item not directly serving this end has been deliberately excluded.

Acknowledgement: Thanks giving is a pleasant task. Any work of this nature however small it may be, needs the help of many heads and hands. The author is highly indebted to Shri Y. R. Chada, Director and Chief Editor, Publications and Information Directorate, CSIR, New Delhi, who kindly gave permission to transfer some of the morphological descriptions of drugs from one of the rare and classical works. "The Indian Pharmaceutical Codex" by Dr. B. Mukherji. Grateful thanks are also due to Ms. Lea Febiger, Philadelphia and Ms. Bailliere Tindall, London.

Shri S. Gopalakrishna Nayak, my colleague in the Department, has as usual rendered valuable help in bringing out this edition. I am gratefully indebted to him. Another colleague Shri H. K. Kakrani, has obliged me by supplying relevant information and I owe him grateful thanks.

I also wish to express my sincere thanks to the following: The Management and Academy of General Education, Manipal, Shri T. Ramesh U. Pai, Registrar, Academy of General Education, Manipal, Dr. Ramdas Pai, Medical Director, KMCH, Manipal, Prof. Dr. A. Krishna Rao, Dean, KMC, Manipal, Prof. Dr. P. K. R. Warrier, Prof. and Head of the Department of Surgery, KMCH, Manipal, (Mrs.) Dr. Malati Chauhan, and Prof. Dr. Devani both of LM College of Pharmacy, Ahmedabad and Prof. Dr. H. Wagner, Director, Instituet fuer Pharmazeutische Arzneimittellehre der Universitaet Muenchen, West Germany.

And finally, Mr. Mohandas Pai, Mr. Satish Pai, Mr. Bhaskar Rao and the friendly staff of Manipal Power Press.

Vijayadashami, 1981   **M. A. Iyengar**

PREFACE   *Fifteenth Edition*

If quality is the way of life, nothing can stop it. Thanks to all concerned.

With gratitude and grateful thanks, I acknowledge the commendable, consistent and continuous support from my good friend Dr. Amit Agarwal, Director (R & D) NATURAL REMEDIES Private Limited, Bangalore.

January, 2012   **M. A. Iyengar**

CONTENTS

DRUGS

OTHER PUBLICATIONS BY THE SAME AUTHOR

HOW TO USE THIS BOOK?

One hundred and twentyfive drugs have been screened through a set proforma. The items of proforma are based on the total knowledge of a drug. The official title, the parts used in medicine,the family to which it belongs, synonyms of different Indian languages, photographs and line diagrams of crude drugs, their morphological descriptions, the chemical or active constituents, chemical tests if any, the actual and existing uses in theraphy and substitutes and adulterants where possible are the features in this proforma. Thus the knowledge about a drug is presented in a nutshell. The drugs are arranged in an alphabetical order.

The actual name (Official Title) is followed by a definition as given in Pharmacopoeia of India and Official or Botanical (Biological) source when it is not an IP Drug, the definition covering the botanical name, part of the plant used with remarks if any, and the plant family. The Latin name of every plant appears with the author's name at the end; but the students need not take particular note of this. Photos of uncommon drugs are provided; as a Chinese saying goes, '1,000 hearings are not that effective as one seeing'. Further, line diagrams have been added in this edition so as to help the students to draw directly from the specimens in their records with the aid of these diagrams. Synonyms available in all the important Indian languages are furnished. A student will understand a drug better in his own mother tongue. Chemical and active consituents of a drug are broadly classified and presented with percentage yield. Names of important constituents are also mentioned under the corresponding group headings. A separate chapter on introductory Phytochemistry gives the simple meanings of words like – alkaloids, glycosides etc., their types and the basic structures. One has to understand this part first, after which one can easily remember the various chemical or active constituents.

Important chemical tests are given where needed and the students are advised to carry out these tests themselves independently in their practical classes. The study of Substitutes and Adulterants of the official drug forms an important aspect of Pharmacognosy and care has been taken to provide this information where available. Further, one more addition in this new edition is the histological details of 5 drugs prescribed for the Final D.Pharm. and these are suitably incorporated. Last but not least, all the important medicinal uses are provided. Meanings of various terminologies are explained in brackets immediately after the concerned word immaterial of the number of times the terms being repeated. In other words, care has been taken to make things for students as easy as possible.

The appendices incorporated at the end will facilitate revision and recapitulation of things studied earlier in the text. An index of genera and species appears at the end.

INTRODUCTION TO ELEMENTARY PHYTOCHEMISTRY

Phytochemistry (Phyton-plant) is the chemistry dealing with plants or plant products or natural products (chemistry of natural products). Natural products comprise different chemical constituents. These chemical constituents may be therapeutically active or inactive. The ones which are active are called active constituents or active principles (alkaloids, glycosides etc.). The inactive ones are called inert chemical constituents (starch, cellulose etc.). Such inert constituents, though they possess no pharmacological or therapeutical activity, are essential for the normal physiological processes.

Active constituents can therefore be defined as chemical constituents which exert even in minute quantities a therapeutic action either on the entire organism or even on a small tissue of the organism. The extraction of these active principles may be very simple like making aqueous infusion, decoction, tincture etc. or may be slightly more elaborate like extracting with various organic solvents and later effecting further separation by employing suitable methods like chromatography etc. Following are the active constituents included in the course:

Alkaloids: Alkaloids are naturally occurring, nitrogenous organic compounds. They are mostly basic in character and exist in plants in the form of salts of inorganic or organic acids. The nitrogen they contain may be a part of the open chain or a part of the ring system (heterocyclic).

It may be worth quoting here another definition of alkaloids given by a well known chemotaxonomist — Professor Hegnauer — "Alkaloids are more or less toxic substances which act primarily on the central nervous system, have a basic character, contain heterocyclic nitrogen, and are synthesised in plants from amino acids or their immediate derivatives. In most cases they are of limited distribution in the plant kingdom".

On the basis of their basic aromatic structures, alkaloids may be classified into the following groups (see Chart 1). It should be mentioned here that only the drugs under discussion and the corresponding types of alkaloids are furnished.
1. Tropane (Belladonna herb, Hyoscyamus and Datura) 2. Indole (Rauwolfia, Ergot etc.) 3. Quinoline (Cinchona) 4. Isoquinoline (Ipecac) 5. Steroid (Kurchi) 6. Phenanthrene (Opium — Morphine) 7. Pyrazole (Withania) 8. Diterpenoid (Aconite).

For detecting alkaloids in phytochemical screening the following general reagents are frequently used: Mayer's, Dragendorff's and Hager's.

Although alkaloids in general are very important therapeutically there are some which are not used in medicine at all. Alkaloids act in small doses mainly on the central or autonomic nervous system. A glance at the various alkaloidal drugs in this book gives an idea that alkaloids are good analgesics, antipyretics, antispasmodics, stimulants, narcotics, sedatives, to mention a few.

Glycosides: Glycosides are naturally occurring organic compounds which yield on hydrolysis a sugar portion and a non-sugar portion referred to as aglycone. The type

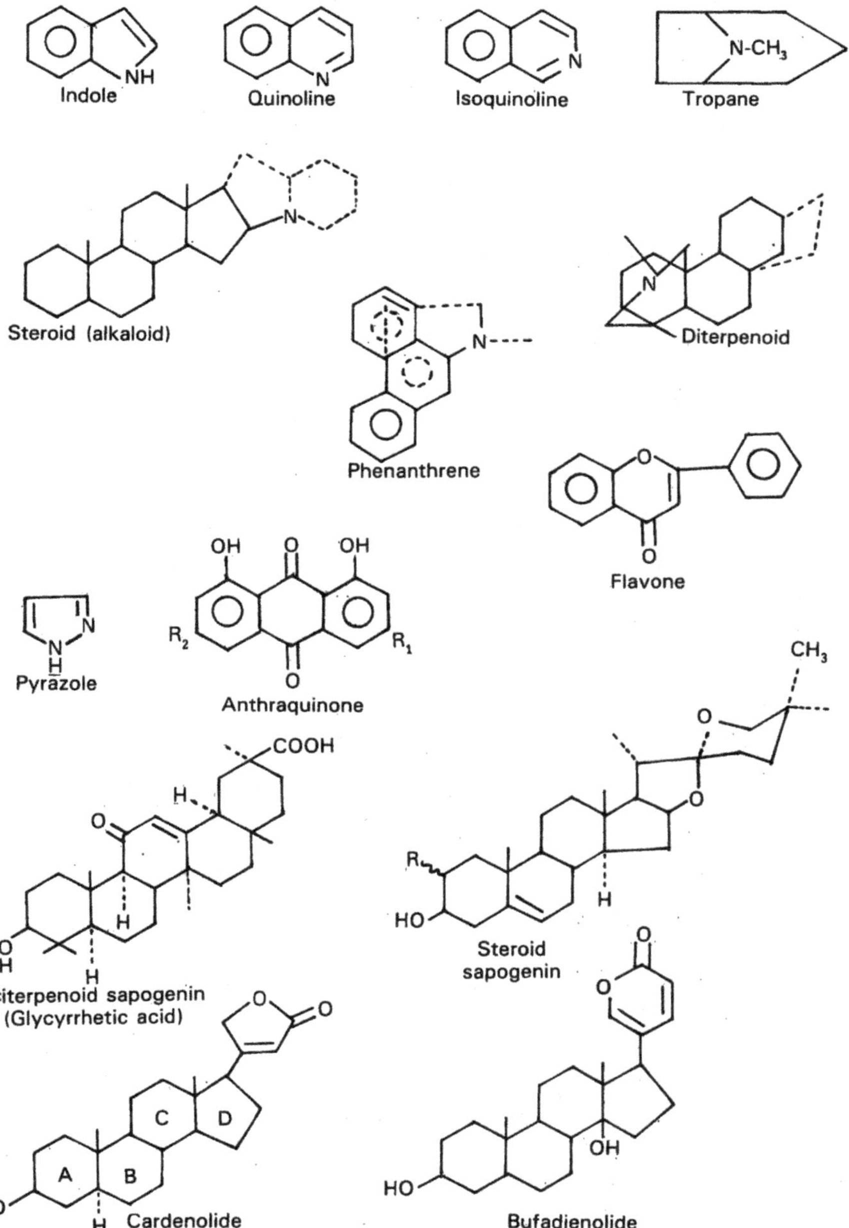

Chart 1: Basic structures of some phytoconstituents

of linkage between the reducing group of sugars and the phenolic hydroxyl or alcoholic group of aglycone is called a 'hemi-acetal' linkage. Glycosides of this type are referred to as O-glycosides which easily undergo hydrolysis. Besides, there are other types like C-glycosides (which do not undergo hydrolysis under normal conditions), N-and S-glycosides. The following types of glycosides are found in the drugs listed in the text. According to the basic structure of the aglycone molecule, glycosides are further grouped as under.

Steroidal (Cardiac) glycosides (eg. Digitalis): Their aglycones have a steroid structure (Chart 1) and are responsible for the specific action (intensity of heart beat is increased and the rate of heart beat is decreased). A lactone ring is attached at C_{17} of the aglycone. Based on the lactone ring, Cardiac glycosides are divided into two groups; if 5 membered lactone ring then Cardenolides – Chart 1 (eg. *Digitalis, Strophanthus etc.)* and if 6 membered lactone ring, then Bufadienolides (Chart 1) or Scilladienolides *(eg. Urginea).* Lactone ring is very important for the therapeutic activity. Removal of lactone ring or even a slight disturbance to the lactone ring means that the activity of the compound is lost. Cardiac glycosides contain a special sugar called digitoxose, though they do carry other sugars like glucose and rhamnose. Very often diuretic action is also associated with steroidal glycosides as they also promote improved circulation of blood through kidneys.

Saponin glycosides (eg. Licorice): The aglycones which result after hydrolysis of the glycosides are called sapogenins. Sapogenins could be either of steroid – of triterpenoid type (Chart 1). Saponin drugs form froth when shaken with water justifying their use in soap industry or as detergents. They do have medicinal values. They are employed for instance as expectorants, emetics, diuretics etc.

Anthracene glycosides (eg. Senna, Aloes): These are very good laxatives. They irritate the mucosa of the gut, mainly of the large intestine. Chemically they are derivatives of anthracene (Chart 1). Anthracene derivatives occur usually in two forms: – the oxidation form (the anthraquinones (Chart 1) and reduced forms (anthrones and anthranols). Anthrones and anthranols are tautomers. Two anthrones may join back to back to form dianthrones. Therapeutically anthraquinones are less milder, anthrones milder than anthranols. Consequently the corresponding glycosides are more active than their aglycones.

Cyanogenetic glycosides (eg. Wild cherry bark): These yield on hydrolysis hydrocyanic acid as one of the products.

Flavonoid glycosides (eg. Licorice): These are mostly yellow pigments present in plants. They are phenolic in nature. They are derivatives of 2 – phenylbenzopyrones (Chart 1). A large number of physiological activities have been attributed to them. Some flavones may act as cardiac stimulants, some strengthen weak capillary blood vessels, some are good diuretics and of late some have proved extremely good against liver damage.

Resinous glycosides (eg. Ipomoea): Some cathartic drugs owe their purgative action to the resin part of the glycoside.

Sugar portion of the glycosides: Sugars present may consist of one molecule of simple sugar like glucose or rhamnose in which case it will be called a monosaccharide, if two monosaccharide units are attached to one another then it is disaccharide and likewise depending on the number of sugar units it may be polysaccharides.

If glucose is the sugar portion of a glycoside, it is then called glucoside, if rhamnose, then rhamnoside and so on. Sugars in the cardiac glycosides are special in that they are 2 – desoxy sugars (Digitoxose).

Although the aglycone is responsible for the attributed therapeutic activity, it is very essential that sugars should also be present for promoting the action (Transport and protective function).

Tannins (eg. Catechu): Tannins are naturally occurring complex organic compounds possessing nitrogen free polyphenols of high molecular weight. They form colloidal solutions with water giving acidic reaction. They also precipitate proteins and alkaloids. The astringent nature of tannins is due to the fact that they can precipitate proteins and render them resistant to enzymatic attack. When applied on a wound or injury, tannins form a protective coating so as to prevent external irritation and thus promote healing. Hydrolysable tannins give blue colour and condensed tannins give green colour with $FeCl_3$ solution.

Volatile Oils (eg. Mentha oil): Volatile oils are volatile principles obtained from plant materials by steam distillation. They possess characteristic odour. The volatile oils (essential oils) differ from fatty or fixed oils in that the former is capable of volatilization, do not leave any spot on the paper, and do not contain glyceryl esters of fatty acids. The active constituents present in volatile oils are terpenes in association with alcohols, phenols, ketone, aldehyde or esters. They have largely carminative action. Some are good appetizers as they can stimulate the secretion of gastric juice. Some volatile oils are good expectorants, diuretics, antiseptics, anthelmintics and antiparasitics, to mention a few.

Lipids: Comprise biosynthetically derived emollients (external applications) and demulcents (internal applications) which are used as mild soothing agents to soften skin or to counteract the irritation of abrasions of skin or of inflamed surfaces. They are present in all parts of plants though rich in seeds and fruits. They serve the function of food storage and energy storage. In commerce and industry, they are used in a number of ways.

Lipids are esters of long chain fatty acids and alcohols. Depending on the type of alcohol, lipids are classified further (a) Fats and Oils – glycerol being the alcohol here (b) Waxes – here alcohols of higher molecular weight (c) Phospholipids with polyhydroxy alcohols.

95% of lipids are made of glycerides whereas the other 5% consist of waxes, sterins, fat soluble vitamins etc., Fats and oils differ only in melting point and the oils are further characterized as non-drying (olive oil), semi-drying (arachis oil, sesame oil) and drying oils (linseed oil). The drying oils are mostly used in the paint, varnish and lacquer industry. Animals also store fat either in fat depots or in liver as in the case of cod and shark and at times in the hairs of sheep (wool), which is a source of lanolin.

A good many oils are edible, some form good ointment bases and a few are good purgatives. Some possess toxic constituents to lower animals and act as anthelmintics.

Waxes are the esters of fatty acids with high molecular weight alcohols (eg. Beeswax).

Gums: These are plant exudates. Chemically they are amorphous polysaccharides. They have protecting and soothing action. Some are good laxatives while others are used in pharmaceutical preparations as emulsifying or suspending agents. Needless to mention, they are also good adhesives.

Resins: Resins are naturally occurring complex organic compounds. Like gums these are also exudates from the tree bark. They are oxidation products of essential oils. Resins are used in wound dressing and for filling the cavities of caries teeth as they melt, when heated, to form an adhesive mass.

Oleo-resins: Resins in homogenous combination with volatile oils (Oil of turpentine). These are good carminatives, disinfectants etc.

Gum-resins: Resins in homogenous combination with gums (Myrrh). These have soothing property.

Oleo-gum-resins: Resins in homogenous mixture with gums and volatile oils (eg. Asafetida).

Balsams: Resins in combination with aromatic acids like Cinnamic — and Benzoic acids (eg. Benzoin).

Some resins like that of *Cannabis* (Hashish) have altogether a different action like-psychotropic, narcotic and sedative.

Bitter principles: Evidently they are bitter to taste. In the real sense they do not form a chemical group but they are an assortment of other active principles like alkaloids, glycosides etc. Because they are able to stimulate the secretion of gastric juice and flow of saliva, they are popular as good appetizers and tonics.

Organic acids: These are present in plants as aliphatic — and aromatic acids. The former are used as mild expectorants, diuretics and laxatives, while the latter are often used as fungistatic in dentistry and as pharmaceutical aids, in general.

Carbohydrates: These comprise largely sugars, starches, cellulose etc. These are widely distributed in plants. Starch finds its use in pharmacy as dusting powder, in the preparation of poultice and as an ingredient of pills. It is also used as a food stuff.

Sugars are not only administered to convalescing patients but are also used as a prophylactic in liver infections and poisons. Further, their useful role in cardiac insufficiency has been reported.

ACACIA

Source: Acacia is the dried exudation from the stem and branches of *Acacia senegal* Willd. and certain other species of *Acacia* (Fam. Leguminosae).

Synonyms and Regional Names: Ben. Hin. Babul; Kan. Gondu; Mal. Karuvelam; San. Vabbula, Babbula; Tam. Karuvelam; Tel. Nallatumma.

Characters: Form – rounded or ovoid tears; Size – variable; Colour – colourless to slight yellowish tint; Fracture – brittle; Fractured surface – glossy; Odour – none; Taste – bland and mucilaginous.

Active Constituents: CARBOHYDRATES – Polysaccharides – Arabin (a mixture of calcium, magnesium and potassium salts of arabic acid), Arabin on hydrolysis gives D – galactose, L-arabinose, L-rhamnose and D-glucuronic acid.

Therapeutical and Pharmaceutical Uses: 1. Demulcent 2. Emulsifying agent 3. Suspending agent 4. Binding agent.

Chemical Tests

1. Solubility: Soluble in water and insoluble in alcohol.
2. A hot aqueous soln. of the gum is acidic.
3. A 10% aqueous soln. of the gum gives with dil. soln. of lead subacetate white precipitate.
4. Test for reducing sugars: Boil a soln. of gum in dil. HCl. Make the resulting soln. alkaline by adding a few ml of caustic soda. When Fehling's soln. is added to the resulting soln. and heated, a red ppt. of cuprous oxide is formed indicating the liberation of reducing sugars.
5. To a boiled soln. of gum in dil. HCl, barium chloride soln. is added when a white ppt. of barium sulphate is not obtained (distinction from Agar).
6. On adding Iodine soln. to an aqueous soln. of gum, no blue or brown colouration is obtained (absence of starch and dextrin).
7. On adding ferric chloride soln. to an aqueous soln. of the gum, no bluish-black colour is produced indicating the absence of tannins.
8. An aqueous soln. of gum is added to 0.5 ml of H_2O_2 soln. and 0.5 ml of alcoholic benzidine (1%). On vigorous shaking a blue colour is produced due to oxidase enzyme (this test however is not be performed in the lab. as it is alleged that benzidine is carcinogenic).

Substitutes and Adulterants: Indian Acacia an inferior quality of gum is obtained from the stems and branches of *Acacia arabica* and is used in place of official drug.

Ghatti gum or Indian gum, an adulterant, is a gummy exudation obtained from the stem of *Anogeissus latifolia* (Combretaceae). The white gum occurs in vermiform or in round tears. This can however be distinguished with lead subacetate test as it gives only slight precipitate.

ACONITE

Source: Aconite is the dried tuberous root of *Aconitum napellus* L. (Fam. Ranunculaceae). It contains not more than 5% of its aerial stems and not less than 0.6% of the alkaloids of aconite, of which not less than 30% consists of aconitine.

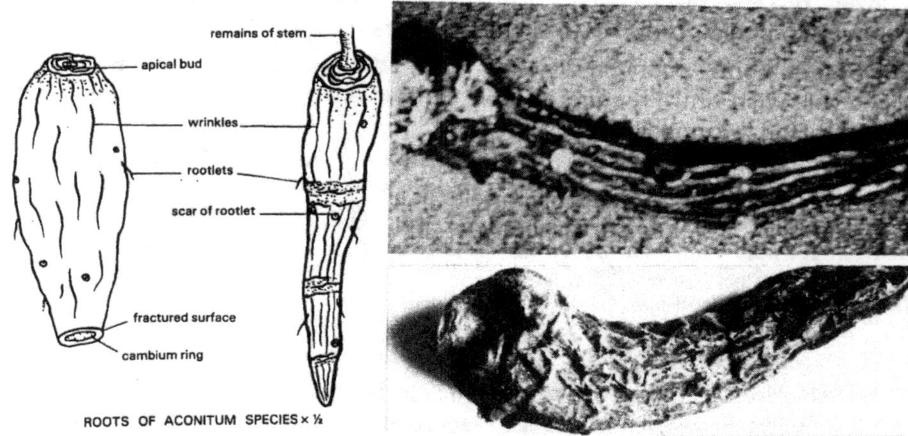

ROOTS OF ACONITUM SPECIES × ½

Synonyms and Regional Names: Monkshood, Ben. Kat-bish; Guj. Ativish, (Vachnag); Hin, Mithazahar, Bachnag; Kan. Ativisha, (Vatsanabhii); Mar. Bachang; San. Visha; Tam. Vashanavi; Tel. Nabhi.

Morphology: Shape – obconical; Size – 4 – 10 cm (l) and from 1 – 3.5 cm (d) at the crown; Colour greyish brown to dark brown; Surface – wrinkled; Fracture – short and Fractured surface – mealy or starchy; Odour – none; Taste – bitter, followed by a persistent tingling sensation. A poisonous drug.

Active Constituents: ALKALOIDS
— Diterpenoid type (easily hydrolysable ester alkaloids of terpenoid structure)
— Aconitine (acetylbenzoylaconine) – Picroaconitine (benzoylaconine)
— Aconine ($C_{25}H_{41}O_9N$) and – in traces Mesaconitine, Hypaconitine, Napelline, Neopelline, Neoline.

Therapeutical and Pharmaceutical Uses:
1. Most poisonous vegetable drug.
2. Tincture aconite is used in neuralgia (pain in the nerve) and rheumatism (pain in the joints or muscles, usually recurrent).
3. Cardiac irritant.
4. In Homeopathic medicines, aconite enjoys a better place as it is very much used in all sorts of fever and catarrhal ailments.
5. Local Analgesic (relieves pain) in liniments (a solution made of an irritant drug in an alcoholic, soapy or oily vehicle meant to be rubbed on the skin as a counter irritant).

8

AGAR

Source: Agar is the dried colloidal concentrate from a decoction of various red algae, particularly species of *Gelidium* and *Pterocladia* (Fam. Gelidiaceae) and *Gracilaria* Fam. Gracilariaceae.

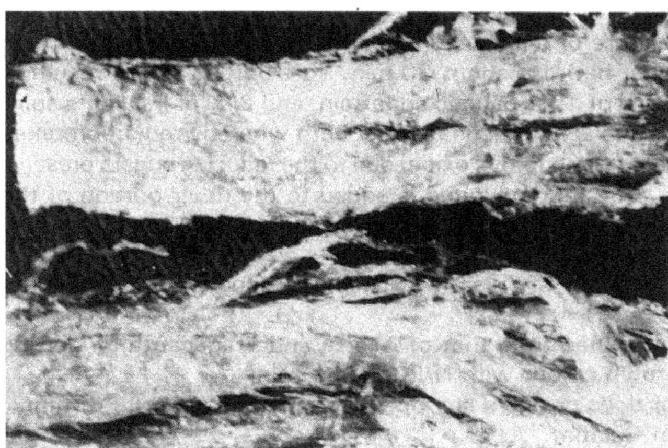

Synonyms
Agar-Agar, Japanese isinglass
Morphology
Form – thin, membranous strips or flattened bands; Colour – colourless, translucent, greyish yellow; Size – 30 – 50 cm(l) and 4 mm(w); Surface – micaceous crinkled; Odour – none; Taste – mucilaginous

Active Constituents: CARBOHYDRATES – Polysaccharides. Heterogenous polysaccharides consisting of two components (a) *Agarose* (70%), a neutral galactose polymer. It is free from sulphate. The gel strength of Agar is due to this component. Agarose also called as Agarobiose is a disaccharide consisting alternate residues of 1, 4-α-linked 1, 3-β-D-glactose and 3,6-anhydro-L-galactose. While the disaccharide unit is called agarobiose or neoagarobiose, the linear chain is called agarose. In otherwords, (agarobiose)$_n$ = agarose. (b) *Agaropectin,* an acidic sulphonated component wherein 1, 3 linked D-galactose and the galacturonic acid (an uronic acid) are partly esterified with sulphuric acid. Agaropectin comprises 90% and more of sulphur. In addition, the sulphate group may also get linked to calcium, magnesium, potassium or sodium.

Therapeutical and Pharmaceutical Uses

1. As a bulk laxative (an agent to induce active movement of the bowels) and in chronic obstipation (unmanageable constipation). Generally it is given in combination with other anthraquinone vegetable drugs.
2. In the preparation of vaginal capsules and suppositories (a cone shaped capsule like structure with the medicine in it, to be introduced into rectum, urethra or vagina).
3. To prepare nutrient media in bacteriological culture.
4. In industrial applications like emulsions, sizing, silk textiles, adhesives and thickening ice cream.

Chemical Tests

1. Solubility test: Agar powder when treated with cold water swells whereas in boiling water dissolves which however on cooling forms gel. (distinction from Acacia and Gelatin).
2. Test for Mucilage: Agar powder takes pink colour on treatment with a soln. of Ruthenium Red. The test is to be performed on a slide and to be observed under a microscope
3. Test for Sugars: A mixture of equal volumes of dil. HCl and aqueous soln. of Agar is heated on water bath for about 30 min. To a portion of the resulting mixture so obtained, 3ml of 10% caustic soda soln. and 2 ml of Fehling's soln. are added and the mixture is heated on a water bath whereby reduction takes place (formation of red ppt. of cuprous oxide) due to the reducing sugars present.
4. Sulphate test: A soln. of barium chloride is added to the other portion of the resulting mixture whereby a white ppt. of barium sulphate is obtained (distinction from Acacia and Tragacanth).
5. On warming a small quantity of Agar in KOH soln. a canary yellow colour is obtained.
6. Powder Agar is distinguished from that of Acacia and Tragacanth by getting a deep crimson to brown colour with N/20 Iodine soln.
7. A 0.2% soln. of Agar does not give any ppt. with an aqueous soln. of tannic acid (distinction from Gelatin).
8. Agar is incinerated to ash. Add dil. HCl and see under the microscope, when skeletons and spongy spicules of diatoms are seen.

ALGINATE

Source: Sodium Alginate or Algin is the purified carbohydrate product obtained from brown algae *Laminaria* species (Fam. Laminariaceae) using dil. alkali.

Nature: Cream coloured powder, forms a viscous and colloidal soln. in water, Odourless and slightly sour in taste.

Chemical composition: CARBOHYDRATE – Sodium salt of alginic acid. Alginic acid is a long chain polyuronide composed of 1 – 4 linkage residues of D-mannuronic acid and L-guluronic acids.

Therapeutical and Pharmaceutical Uses

1. In cosmetics 2. In dermatological preparations. 3. In dental preparations
4. In adhesive paste 5. In textile industry 6. As a general emulsifier
7. In food industry.

ALOES

Source: Aloes is the dried juice of the leaves of *Aloe barbadensis* Miller known in commerce as Curacao aloes or of *Aloe perryi* Baker – Socotrine and Zanzibar aloes or of *A. ferox Miller* or its hybrids – Cape aloes, all belonging to Fam. Liliaceae.

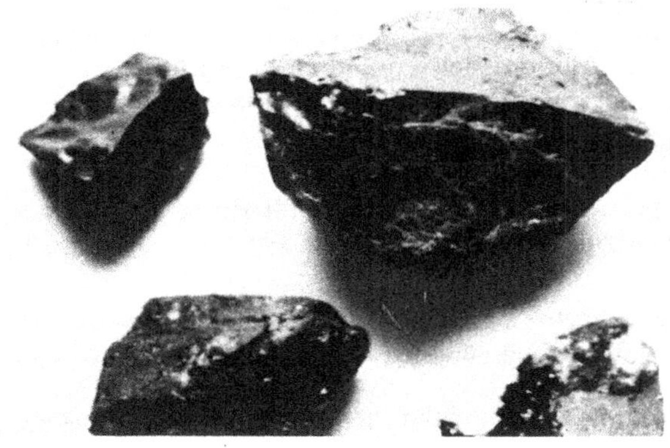

Synonyms and Regional Names

Ben. Ghertokumari
Guj. Kumarpathu
Hin. Musabbar
Kan. Lolirasa
Mal. Kumari, (Kathavazha)
Mar. Khorphad
San. Ghirtakumar
Tam. Kariabolam
Tel. Musambaram

General Morphology: Form – irregular mass; Colour – dark chocolate brown to black; Surface – dull, opaque with slightly vitreous appearance; Fracture – brittle; Odour – characteristic; Taste – bitter and unpleasant. All the 4 commercial forms are compared here below for their morphological characters.

Macroscopic Characters

	Curacao	*Cape*	*Socotrine*	*Zanzibar*
Colour	Yellowish brown to chocolate brown	Dark brown to greenish brown	Yellowish brown to dark brown	Light blue
Form	Hepatic or livery	Vitreous or glassy	Same as Curacao............	
Texture	Opaque	Glassy	Same as Curacao............	
Fracture	Waxy	Brittle	Porous	Waxy
Odour	Iodoform odr.	Rhubarb Odr.	Characteristic	
Taste	All bitter and unpleasant........................			

Active Constituents

GLYCOSIDES — Anthracene glycosides (11 to 40%)
— Barbaloin or Aloin, a C glycoside (not easily hydrolysable with dil. acids and the linkage between the sugar and the aglycone is through C-C)
Isobarbaloin (+ + + Curacao, + Cape and – in the other two)
— Aloinosides A and B (only in cape aloes,-O-glycosides) – glycosides of barbaloin.

These are stereoisomers and are barbaloin-11-O-α-L-rhamnosides or simply
O-rhamnosides of barbaloin.
RESINS (resinotannol + cinnamic acid or coumaric acid).

Therapeutical and Pharmaceutical Uses: 1. Laxative.   2. Used externally for *Ulcus cruris* (a type of ulcer), eczema and burns.   3. As a bitter substance.   4. Aloes have found very many new uses in cosmetics: as a moisture base cleanser, skin toner, night cream, hand and body lotion, hair conditioner, all purpose cream, shampoo, eye lotion as a post operative treatment and also in dental surgery.

Note: Contraindicated in case of pregnancy and during menstruation.

Chemical Tests: Preparation of test solution: 1g of aloes is boiled in 100 ml of water. On cooling, 1g of Kieselguhr is added, stirred and filtered. Filtrate is used for the tests —

1. *Borax test for Anthranol:* (Schonteten's Reaction) 0.5g of borax is heated with 10 ml of test soln. Green coloured fluorescence is seen which is due to aloe-emodin anthranol.
2. *Bromine test:* Heavy yellow ppt. of tetrabromaloin is formed when equal volumes of bromine soln. and test soln. are mixed.
3. *Nitrous acid test for Isobarbaloin:* To 5 ml of test soln. equal volume of sodium nitrite soln. and a few drops of dil. acetic acid are added whereby pink or purplish colour is produced (negative in Zanzibar and Socotrine aloes because of the absence of isobarbaloin).
4. *Nitric acid test:* Based on the presence of Isobarbaloin. Add 2 ml of HNO_3 to a 5 ml soln. of Aloes and observe the colour. A brown colour changing immediately to green – Cape aloes, a deep brownish red – Curacao aloes, a pale brownish yellow – Socotrine aloes and finally a yellowish brown colour – Zanzibar aloes.
5. *Klunge's Isobarbaloin test (Cupraloin test):* Dilute the test soln. by adding equal volume of water in the proportion of 1:1 and to this add a drop of saturated copper sulphate solution + 1g NaCl + 10 ml 90% alcohol. Observe the colour. Wine red colour persists for a long time – Curacao aloes; feeble wine red colour changing soon to yellow – Cape aloes. No colour is obtained in the other two varieties as they do not contain isobarbaloin.
6. *Modified Borntrager's test or modified anthraquinone test:* To 0.1g of the drug Aloes, 5 ml of 5% soln. of ferric chloride and 5 ml dil. HCl are added and boiled on a water bath for 5 minutes. After cooling, the mixture is extracted with an organic solvent like benzene in a separating funnel. The benzene layer is now shaken with an equal volume of dil. ammonia whereby a pinkish red colour is formed in ammoniacal layer.

Substitutes and Adulterants: The East African aloes namely the Socotrine aloes and Zanzibar aloes are inferior varieties and they can be easily distinguished both chemically and morphologically as mentioned above.

AMLA

Source: Amla consists of the fresh or dried fruit of *Emblica officinalis* Linn./*Phyllanthus emblica* Linn. (Fam. Euphorbiaceae).

Synonyms and Regional Names: Ben. Amla, Amlaki; Guj. Amla; Hin. Amla, Aonla; Kan. Nellikai; Mal. Amlakam; Mar. Anoli, Anvala; San. Amlika; Tam. Nellikai; Tel. Amlakamu.

Morphology: Type of fruit-Drupe (tricarpellary); Colour – pale green to yellow and pink when ripe; Form – globose, spherical, fleshy, 6 grooved; Size – 1.3 to 1.6 cm(d), mesocarp – fleshy and edible and endocarp stony; Odour – none; Taste – pleasantly sour.

Active Constituents: TANNINS (13 of them), PHYLLEMBELIN
– Gallic acid, Ellagic acid and Glucose
Rich source of PECTINS and VITAMIN C (600-921 mg/100 g).

Therapeutical and Pharmaceutical Uses: 1. Liver tonic 2. As an aperient (a gentle purgative) 3. In the treatment of jaundice, dyspepsia and cough 4. Cooling, diuretic, astringent and in biliousness 5. It is one of the ingredients of 'Triphala' 6. Richest known source of Vitamin C (ascorbic acid)—Antiscorbutic (counteracting scurvy – disease due to deficiency of ascorbic acid) 7. Antibacterial and Antifungal 8. A mild cerebral depressant 9. Antispasmodic 10. Used in gastritis syndrome to antagonize gastric acid secretions.

ARACHIS OIL

Source: Arachis Oil is a fixed oil obtained by expression from the seeds of the cultivated varieties of *Arachis hypogaea* Linn (Fam. Leguminosae).

Synonyms and Regional Names: Pea nut, Earth nut, Ground nut. Ben. Chineebadam; Guj. Bhoising; Hin. Munghphali; Kan. Mal. Nela Kadale; Mar. Bhuichana; San. Buchanaka; Tam. Vevakadalai; Tel. Veerusanagalu.

Nature: Arachis oil is a non-drying oil; Colour – almost colourless or yellowish; Form – liquid; Odour – nut like; Taste – bland.

Active Constituents: LIPIDS – Mixture of glycerides.
– Oleic, Linoleic, Palmitic, Stearic, Archidic, Behenic and Lignoceric acids.

Therapeutical and Pharmaceutical Uses
1. As a solvent for intramuscular injection 2. As a pharmaceutical aid 3. As a food oil 4. A valuable lubricant 5. In the preparation of soaps.

ARJUNA

Source: Arjuna is the dried bark of *Terminalia arjuna* W. et. A. (Fam. Combretaceae).

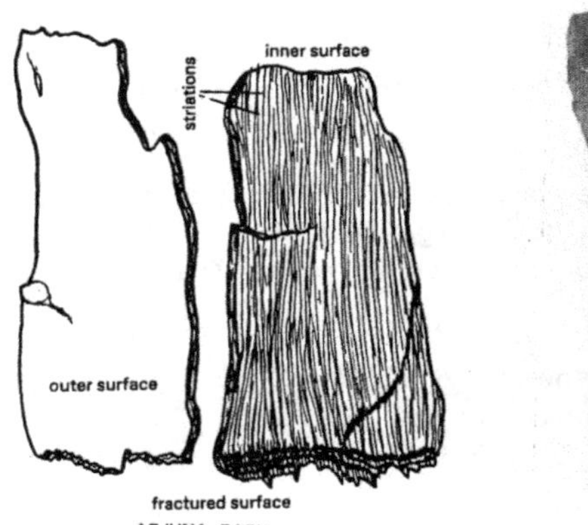

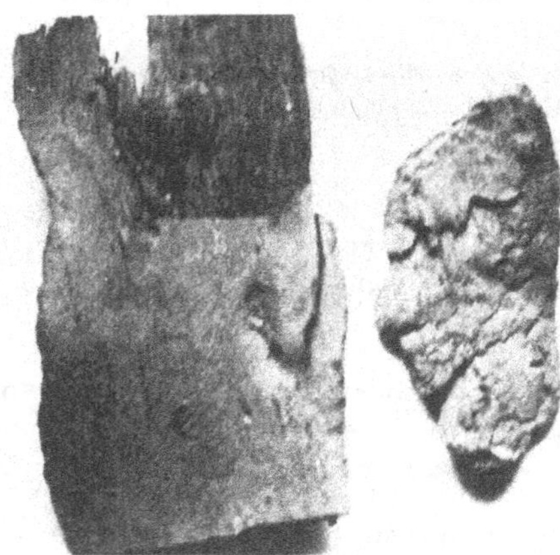

Synonyms and Regional Names: Arjun tree, Ben, Arjun; Guj. Arjun; Hin. Anjan, Arjan; Kan. Holematti; Mal. Venmarutti; Mar. Arjun; San. Arjuna; Tam. Attumarudu, Marudampattai; Tel. Tellamaddicittu.

Morphology: Shape – Flat or slightly curved; Size – around 15 cm(l), 10 cm(b) and 1 cm(t); Colour – ash coloured on the outerside but reddish and striated on the inner side; Surface – more or less smooth; Fracture – fibrous; Odour – none and Taste – astringent.

Active Constituents: 1. TANNINS (12%) – mainly pyrocatechol tannins.
2. Large quantities of CALCIUM SALTS and small traces of ALUMINIUM and MAGNESIUM SALTS.
3. ARJUNGLUCOSIDES, phytosterols, organic acids and organic esters, sugars, colouring matter etc.
4. Responsible for the diuretic property of Arjuna is a saponin like substance.

Therapeutical and Pharmaceutical Uses

1. Mild diuretic (increases the flow of urine).
2. Astringent (arrests discharges or secretions).
3. Cooling, tonic and febrifuge (a drug which reduces fever).
4. Reported to give beneficial effects in ischaemic heart disease.

Substitutes and Adulterants: In commerce, *T. tomentosa* is sold sometimes as *T. arjuna.* Some of the active constituents present in arjuna like tannins are also present here and therefore this is used sometimes in place of arjuna. One can however distinguish the bark from that of the official drug as the bark measures 30 cm in length, 3 cm in thickness and 8 cm in width. Outer surface is again distinct in being rough with cracks and fissures and dark brown colour. Even the fracture being granular and laminated in parts is different from that of arjuna.

ARTEMISIA

Source: Artemisia is obtained from the unexpanded flower heads of *Artemisia cina* Berg and *A. maritima* Linn. (Fam. Compositae).

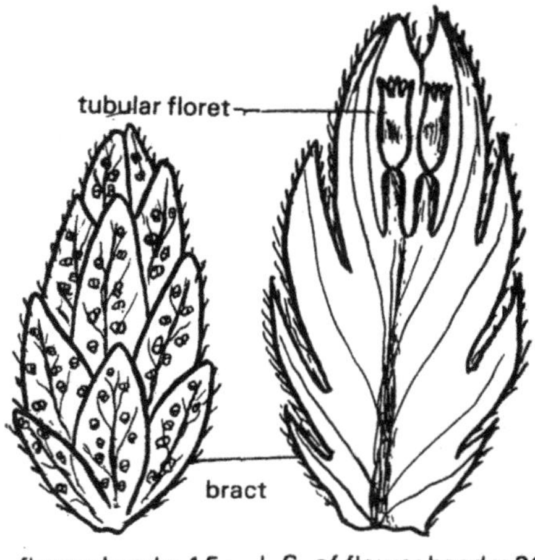

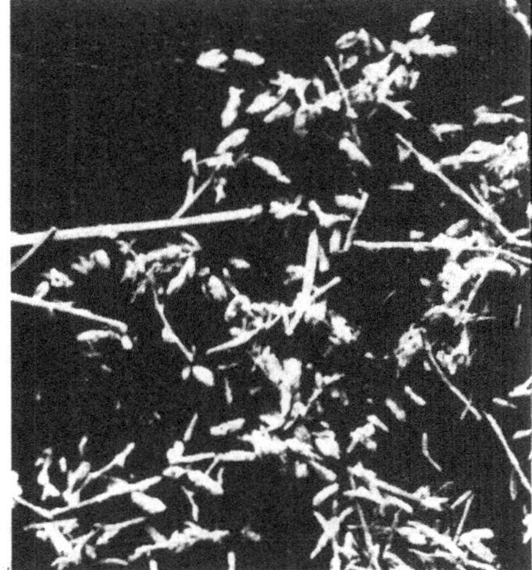

Synonyms and Regional Names: Wormseed, Levant Wormseed, Santonica, Flores Cinae, Guj. Chhuvariajamoda; Hin. Kirmala; Mar. Kiramoniova; San. Chauhara.

Morphology: Type of Inflorescence — cápitulum (the smallest inflorescence known), Size — 1.5 to 4 mm(l). The flower head consists of an involucre of 16 bracts which encloses 2 to 5 immature florets. Form of bract — tongue shaped and bears numerous trichomes both covering and glandular. Covering trichome-convoluted like a worm, unicellular, long, thin walled and in groups giving an appearance of a cottony mass, Glandular trichomes — short with biseriate stalk of two cells and a biseriate head of 4 cells. A bladder like covering of cuticle may be seen around each head. Florets — the immature tubular florets are situated at the top of the elongated axis of the inflorescence. Each floret is elongated and shows 5 teeth of the gamopetalous corolla enclosing 5 syngenesious anthers and stigma. Ovary is inferior; Colour — yellowish green to brown; Odour — strong and aromatic; Taste — bitter and camphoraceous.

Active Constituents

TERPENOIDS — Sesquiterpene
      — Santonin, a crystalline bicyclic sesquiterpene lactone
      — β-Santonin, an isomer though weak in action
      — Pseudosantonin, devoid of any anthelmintic action

VOLATILE OIL — Cineole, Artemisin.

Therapeutical and Pharmaceutical Use: Anthelmintic (expulsion of worms from the stomach) — Vermifuge — chiefly round and thread worms [but not *Taenia* (tape worm)] are expelled but not killed.

ASAFOETIDA

Source: Asafoetida (Asafetida) is the oleo-gum-resin obtained by incising the living rhizomes and roots of *Ferula asafoetida (F. foetida* Regal) (Fam. Umbelliferae).

Synonyms and Regional Names: Devil's dung, Ben. Hing; Guj. Hing; Hin. Heeng; Kan. Hingu; Mar. Hing; San. Hinguka; Tam. Perungayam; Tel. Inguva.

Morphology: Commercial Asafoetida occurs in two forms: 1. Tears either in round or flattened forms. Size – 1 to 3 cm(d); Colour – dull yellow, greyish white or at times reddish brown. 2. Masses – most common form, tears agglutinate to form masses and also contain impurities like piece of fruit, root etc. Surface – rough in general; Fracture – brittle; Odour – strong, alliaceous (garlic smell) and persistent; Taste – alliaceous, bitter and acrid.

Active Constituents

VOLATILE OIL (4 – 20%) – isobutyl propanyl disulphide, also responsible for the bad smell.

RESINS (40 – 65%) – free Asaresinotannol and as well in combination with Ferulic acid.

GUM (25%)

The drug contains no free umbelliferone unlike Galbanum another species of *Ferula.* But then because of the presence of free Ferulic acid, asafetida answers combined Umbelliferone test.

Therapeutical and Pharmaceutical Uses

1. As a carminative (relieves excessive collection of gas in the stomach).
2. As an expectorant [an agent that promotes the removal of catarrhal (discharge from the mucous membrane) matter and phlegm from the bronchial tubes].
3. As an antispasmodic (a drug that counteracts a sudden, violent, involuntary muscular contraction).
4. As a laxative (which induces active movement of bowels).

Chemical Tests

1. Asafoetida forms an emulsion with water; with alcohol it is partially soluble.
2. When triturated with water, it forms yellowish orange emulsion.
3. On addition of H_2SO_4 to the freshly fractured surface, red or reddish brown colour is produced which changes to violet when washed with water.
4. Addition of 50% nitric acid to the fractured surface results in green colour.
5. 0.2 g of the powdered asafoetida is added to 5 ml of 90% alcohol and boiled for 2 min. Cool and filter. To this is added 0.5 ml of 10% ammonia soln. No blue fluorescence is obtained because of the absence of free umbelliferone.
6. *Combined Umbelliferone Test:* Triturate the drug (if in tear form) with sand. Boil 0.5 g of the drug with 3 ml of HCL + 3 ml of water for 5 to 10 min. Filter and to the filtrate add an equal volume of alcohol and excess of strong soln. of ammonia. A blue fluorescence is produced becasue of the presence of combined umbelliferone.

ASOKA

Source: Asoka consists of the dried stem bark of *Saraca indica* L. (Fam. Leguminosae).

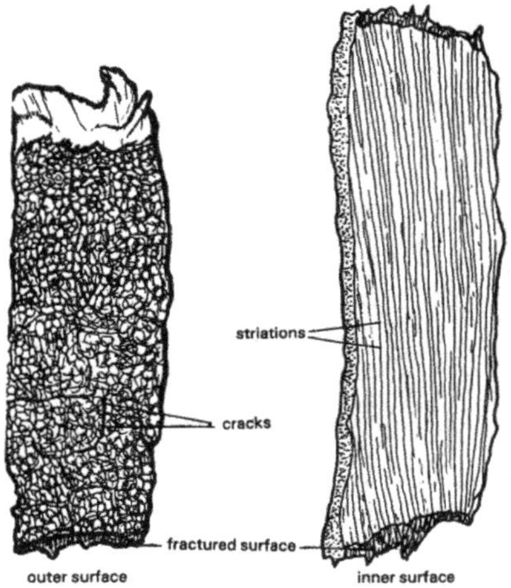

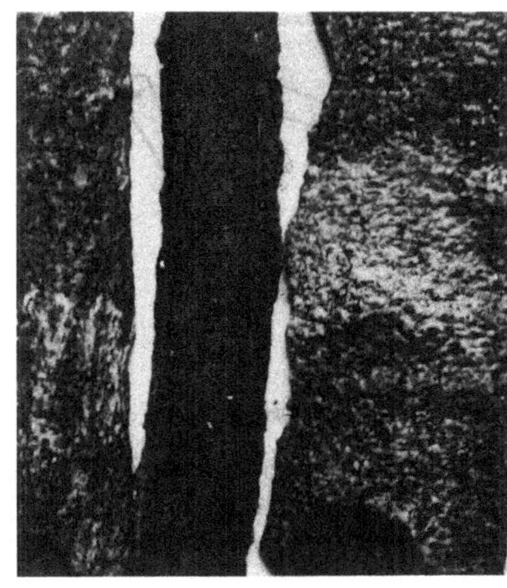

Synonyms and Regional Names: Ben. Asoka; Guj. Ashoka; Hin. Ashoka; Kan. Asoka; Mal. Asokam; Mar. Ashok; San. Anganapriya, Shokanashaka; Tam. Asoka; Tel. Asokumu,

Morphology: Form – Market sample usually varies in form from flat to channelled. Outer surface – dark, rough and with cracks, inner surface – red, smooth with striations; Fracture – very tough; Odour – none and Taste – astringent.

Active Constituents:
TANNINS and crystalline glycosides in traces.

Therapeutical and Pharmaceutical Uses

1. Highly astringent.
2. A very good household remedy for uterine disorders, especially for menorrhoegia (excessive menstruation), Leucorrhoea (a whitish discharge from the vagina), internal piles and dysentery.
3. Ashoka is used in 55 drug preparations (Kapoor & Mitra).

Substitutes and Adulterants: Ashoka tree means to a common man the tall slender, green and decorative trees of *Polyalthia longifolia* (Annonanceae) and as such not related in any way to *Saraca indica.*

ASWAGANDHA

Source: Aswagandha consists of dried roots and stem bases of *Withania somnifera* Dun. (Fam. Solanaceae).

Synonyms and Regional Names: Withania root, Winter cherry, Ben. Aswagandha; Guj. Asoda; Hin. Asgand; Kan. Hirimaddina Gadde, Amakire; Mal. Amukkiram; Mar. Askandha, Kanchuki; San. Ashwagandha; Tam. Ammukkarankilangu; Tel. Penneru.

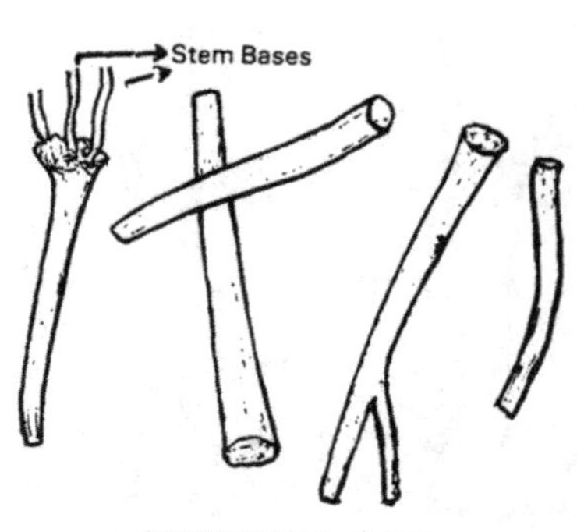

ASWAGANDHA ROOTS

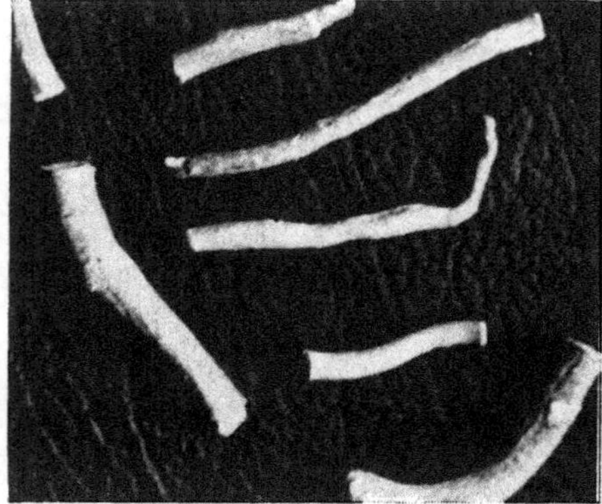

Morphology: Form – straight, unbranched and cylindrical; Colour – buff to greyish yellow with longitudinal wrinkles; Fracture – short and fractured surface cream coloured. Stem bases are also seen. Odour – strong and Taste – slightly bitter.

Active Constituents:

ALKALOIDS – Pyrazole alkaloids – Withasomnine – withanine – cuscohygrine – – anahygrine – anaferine.

STEROIDAL LACTONES – Withaferin A (o.2%), – Withanolides.

Therapeutical and Pharmaceutial Uses.

1. Sedative (reduces excitement, pain etc.).
2. Tonic, Stimulant, Aphrodisiac (arouses sexual desire) and for toning up the uterus.
3. Withaferin is a bacteriostatic and antitumerous agent.
4. Aswagandha is used in 109 drug preparations (Kapoor & Mitra).

BAEL

Source: Bael consists of the entire unripe or half ripe fruit of *Aegle marmelos* L. Corr. (Fam. Rutaceae).

Synonyms and Regional Names: Bengal quince, Ben. Bael; Guj. Bilvaphal; Hin. Bel; Kan. Bil patre; Mal. Koovlam; Mar. Bel, San. Bilva; Tam. Vilvam; Tel. Bilvamu.

Morphology: Type of Fruit – Berry; Colour – green (unripe) and yellowish brown (ripe); Size – 7.5 to 20 cm(d); Shape – sub-globose; Surface – smooth but hard and woody; Epicarp – 3 mm(t). Pulp consisting of mesocarp and endocarp is pale red in colour. Seeds – numerous and a sticky mucilage surrounds the seeds. Odour – slightly aromatic and Taste – mucilaginous.

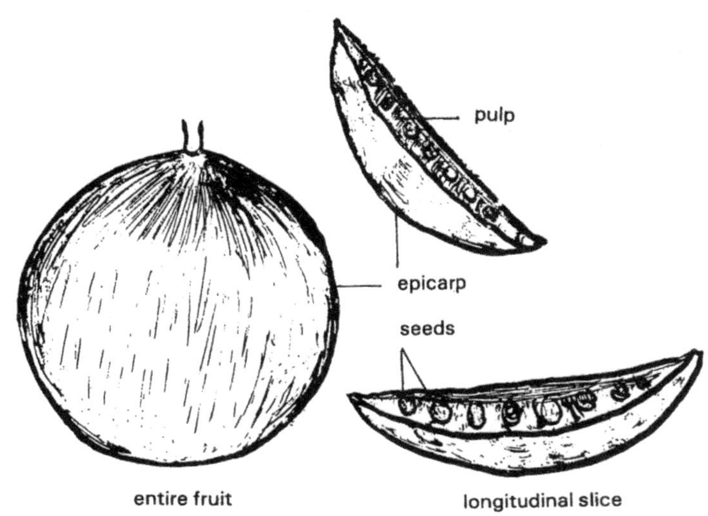

BAEL × ½

Active Constituents: FUROCOUMARINS – Marmelosin (0.03 – 0.4%) TANNINS (20%), REDUCING SUGARS (3.7%)

Therapeutical and Pharmaceutical Uses

1. In cases of chronic diarrhoea (frequent evacuation of watery faeces) and dysentery (evacuation of liquid, bloody and mucous stools).
2. The 'sherbat' made out of the ripe pulp has as well a cooling effect.
3. Bael is used in 60 different drug preparations (Kapoor & Mitra).

Substitutes and adulterants: Bael trees are grown in almost all the important temples in India. Being very common, the fruits are not subjected to any serious adulteration or substitution. However, occasionally the fruits of *Garcinia mangostana* (Mangosteen fruits) Fam. Guttiferae, and Wood apple fruits – *Feronia elephantum* Fam. Rutaceae are substituted. Mangosteen fruits have darker rind to which the pulp does not adhere firmly. Wood apple fruits show roughness on the external side and are 5 lobed and 1 – celled internally.

BAHERA

Source: Bahera consists of the dried fruit of *Terminalia belerica* Roxb. (Fam. Combretaceae). It is one of the constituents of 'TRIPHALA'.

Synonyms and Regional Names: Ben. Bahera, Bohera; Guj. Beheda; Hin. Mar. Bahera, Behara; Kan. Santhi, Tare; Mal. Thani; Tam. Akkam, Tanri; Tel. Tadi, Tandra.

Morphology: Type of fruit – drupe; Form – ovoid or obovoid; Colour – grey and velvety; Size – 2.5 cm(l); Odour – none and Taste – acrid and astringent.

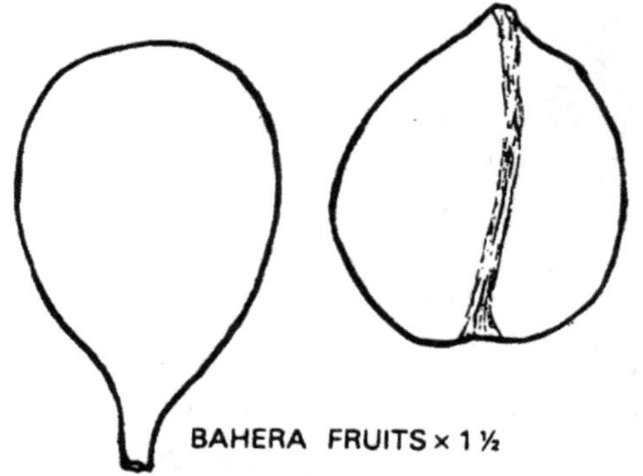

Active Constituents: TANNINS (17%) – gallic acid – ellagic acid – ethylgallate – galloyl glucose, chebulagic acid – mannitol – glucose – galactose – fructose – rhamnose. FIXED OIL (38%) – Palmitic, stearic, oleic and linoleic acids.

Therapeutical and Pharmaceutical Uses: 1. Astringent, tonic and antiseptic 2. In the treatment of diarrhoea and dysentery 3. Purgative 4. Antidiabetic.

BALSAM OF TOLU

Source: Tolu Balsam is a solid or semi-solid balsam obtained by incision from the trunk of *Myroxylon balsamum* L. Harms. (Fam. Leguminosae). It contains not less than 35% and not more than 50% of total balsamic acids, calculated with reference to the dry alcohol soluble matter.

Characters: Colour – Brownish yellow to brown; Odour – aromatic (vanilla smell); Solubility – Insoluble in water; soluble in alcohol, ether, chloroform etc.

Active Constituents

RESINS (80%) – Resin alcohols combined with Cinnamic – and Benzoic acids. (Resin esters of Tolu resinotannols).
VOLATILE OIL (7.8%) – Benzyl benzoate
FREE ORGANIC ACIDS – Cinnamic acid (2 – 15%), Benzoic acid (8%).

Therapeutical and Pharmaceutical Uses

1. As an expectorant (an agent that promotes the removal of catarrhal matter and phlegm from the bronchial tubes). 2. Flavouring agent 3. As an antiseptic.

Chemical Tests

1. An alcoholic solution of the drug is acidic.
2. Green colouration is obtained by adding ferric chloride soln. to alcoholic (90%) soln. of Tolu.
3. Bring to boil 1 g of Tolu balsam in 5 ml. water, filter and heat the filtrate with 30 mg of $KMnO_4$. Benzaldehyde odour can be noted.

Adulterant: Colophony as an adulterant is detected by cupric acetate reaction (see Colophony).

Note: It is reported that modern samples show an increase in benzoic acid content, a decreased cinnamic acid content and the absence of benzyl cinnamate. Some contained additional unreported constituents like cinnamaldehyde and benzyl alcohol. (Planta Med. 1979. 35(1), 61).

BANAFSHA

Source: Banafsha consists of the above ground herb including flowers of *Viola odorata* Linn. and *V. pilosa* (Blume) (Fam. Violaceae).

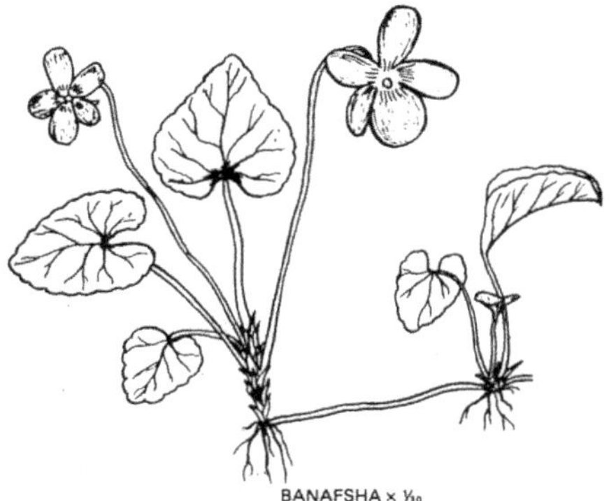

BANAFSHA × ⅟₁₀

Morphology: Small pubescent herb, upto 50 cm(h); Flowers – showy and axillary and emit sweet aroma.

Active Constituents: (in flowers) ALKALOID – Isoquinoline type – Violine. VOLATILE OIL – Ketones present are responsible for characteristic smell of flowers. SAPONIN – a Saponin like substance has been reported from the rootstock.

Therapeutical and Pharmaceutical Uses: 1. Expectorant, diaphoretic, antipyretic and diuretic. 2. The flowers are emollient and demulcent. 3. Emetic (violine). 4. It has a great demand in Unani medicine.

BAVCHI

Source: Bavchi consists of the dried fruits of *Psoralea corylifolia* L. (Fam. Leguminosae).

Synonyms and Regional Names: Malaya tea, Bawchang seed; Ben. Latakasturi; Guj. Bavachi; Hin. Babchi; Kan. Bavuchige; Mal. Karkolari; Mar. Babchi; San. Sugandha Kantak; Tam. Karbogarisi; Tel. Baavanchelu Kala-ginja.

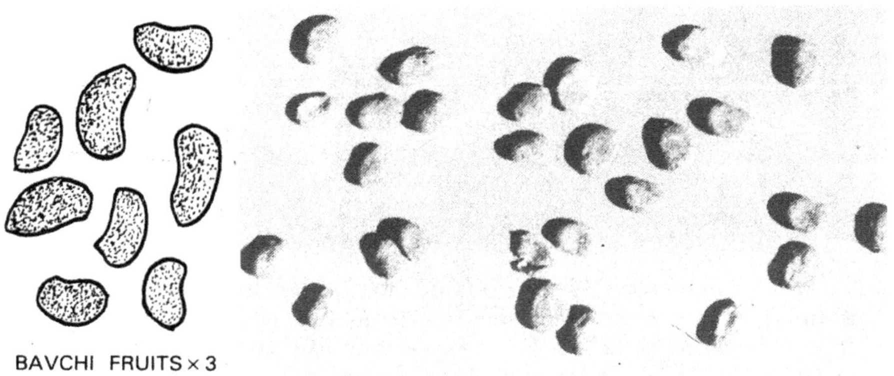

BAVCHI FRUITS × 3

Morphology: Type of fruit – Indehiscent one seeded pod; Form – ovoid-oblong, somewhat compressed, glabrous, mucronate, closely pitted, the oily and sticky pericarp adhering to seeds; Colour – dark chocolate to almost black or dull black. Odourless but on chewing the seed emits a pungent odour and has a bitter, unpleasant and acrid taste.

Active Constituents

ESSENTIAL OIL (0.05 – 0.25%) — Limonene – elemene – Caryophyllene – Oxide – 4 terpineol – linalool – geranyl acetate Bakuchiol (a phenol)

FIXED OIL (about 10%)

FUROCOUMARINS — Psoralen, Isopsoralen, Psoralidin, Isopsoralidin, Corylifolin and Corylifolinin

FLAVONOIDS — Bavachinin (flavanone) – Psoralenol (isoflavone) – Bavachromanol (chalcone) and Isoneobavachalcone.

Therapeutical and Pharmaceutical Uses

1. Leucoderma (Vitiligo) of non syphilitic origin (due to fixed oil and furocoumarins).
2. Antibacterial and antifungal (Essential Oil).
3. Anti-inflammatory, antipyretic and analgesic (bavachinin).
4. Anthelmintic, diuretic and diaphoretic.

BEESWAX

Source: Yellow beeswax is the purified wax from the honey comb of the bee *Apis dorsata* L. and possibly other species of *Apis* (Fam. Apidae). White beeswax is however prepared from yellow beeswax by bleaching with certain chemicals.

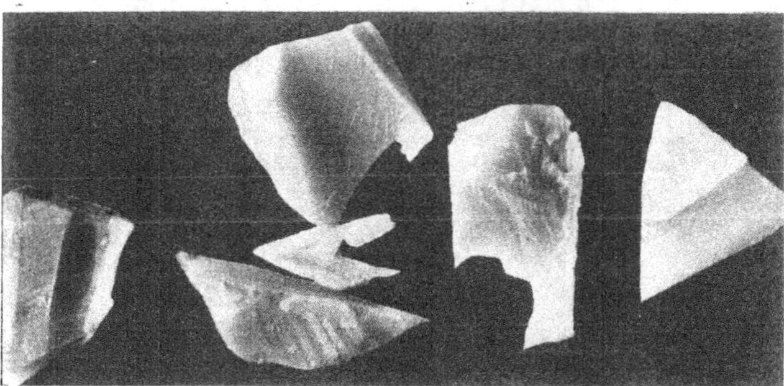

Synonyms and Regional Names

Beeswax
Ben. Mom
Guj. Min
Hin. Mom
Kan. Mena
Mal. Mezhuku
Mar. Mena
San. Madhujan
Tam. Mellugu
Tel. Mainam

Characters: Colour – White or Yellow; Fracture – brittle and granular; Solubility – soluble in chloroform, ether and in both essential and fatty oils, but insoluble in water. M.P. 62° to 64°. Ref. Index to 80°, 1,4380 to 1,4420, Sp. Gravity 0.958 to 0.970. Odour – honeylike, Taste – Waxy.

Chemical (active) Constituents: LIPIDS – Wax

Myricyl palmitate (80%)

Wax-acids – Cerotic acid (15%)

Therapeutical and Pharmaceutical Uses: 1. As a pharmaceutical aid 2. In the preparation of plasters, ointments and polishes.

Chemical Test: Fats, fixed oils and resins are often added to beeswax. These can be detected by the following test:

Saponification Cloud Test: Boil 0.5 g beeswax for 10 min. in 8 ml of 10% Sodium hydroxide soln. Make up the original volume, filter through glass wool and acidify with HCl. If fats, fatty acids or resins are present a ppt. is formed. Fats may be saponified by boiling with aq. sodium hydroxide. Waxes are saponified by strong alcoholic potash, but are practically unaffected by aq. alkali.

BELLADONNA HERB

Source: Belladonna Herb consists of the leaves or leaves and other aerial parts, of *Atropa belladonna* L. or *A. acuminata* Royl ex Lindley (Fam. Solanaceae), or a mixture of both species, collected when the plants are in flower and dried. It contains not less than 0.3% of the alkaloids of Belladonna Herb, calculated as hyoscyamine.

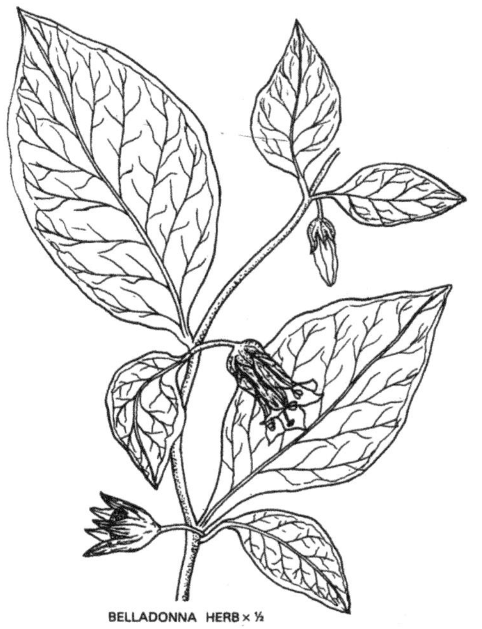

BELLADONNA HERB × ½

Synonyms and Regional Names
Deadly night shade,
Belladonna leaf
Ben. Yebruj
Hin. Sagangur, Angurshefa

Morphology
Leaves: Type – simple;
Form – broadly ovate;
Colour – yellowish – green;
Arrangement – alternate;
arranged in pairs on the
upper stems, each pair with
a large and a small leaf;
Size – 5 to 25 cm(l) 2.5 –
12 cm(b); Margin – entire;
Apex – acuminate;
Surface – slightly hairy.

Petiole – petiolate, petiole 4 cm(l); Flowers: Colour – purple; Size – 2.5 cm(l) 1.2 cm(w); Arrangement of flowers – born singly upon short, druping pedicels arising in the axils of the pairs of leaves; Corolla – campanulate; Calyx – 5 lobed, Stamens-5, epipetalous; Ovary – superior, bilocular with numerous ovules and axile placentation. Fruit; Colour – green to dark purplish black, Type – berry.

Active Constituents: ALKALOIDS – Tropane alkaloids (0.2 – 0.5%) L – hyoscyamine (90%), D,L – hyoscyamine (Atropine), Scopolamine (10%), Apoa-tropine(+), Belladonnine(+).

Therapeutical and Pharmaceutical Uses

1. Mydriatic (dilation of the pupil).
2. Antispasmodic (a drug that counteracts a sudden, violent, involuntary muscular contraction).
3. Antimuscarinic (acts peripherally to produce parasympathetic inhibition).
4. Antisialagogue (a drug that inhibits the flow of excess saliva).
5. Cerebral sedative (reduces excitement).

Vitali Test: A drop of fuming HNO_3 is added to a small portion of an extract of any Solanaceous drugs like species of *Atropa,* Hyoscyamus and *Datura* of the tropane alkaloids themselves and then evaporated to dryness on a water bath. Thereafter it is cooled and on addition of 2 drops of 5% alcoholic potassium hydroxide solution, purple colour is formed indicating the presence of tropane alkaloids.

Substitutes and Adulterants: Belladonna is compared alongwith two common adulterants

Name	Atropa belladonna (Fam. Solanaceae)	Phytolacca decandra (Phytolaccaceae)	Ailanthus glandulosa (Simaroubaceae)
Leaf	Simple	Simple	Compound
Shape	Broadly ovate	Lanceolate	Triangularly ovate
Epidermal cells	Wavy wall with striated cuticle	Straight walls	Straight walls with strongly striated cuticle
Trichomes	Multicellular covering and glandular trichome	Absent	White, unicellular lignified covering trichomes
Stomata	Cruciferous	Ranunculaceous	Ranunculaceous
Calcium oxalate Crystals	Sandy balls	Acicular raphides	Cluster crystals

BELLADONNA ROOT

Source: Belladonna Root is the dried root or root and root-stock of *Atropa belladonna* L. or *A. acuminata* Royl ex Lindley (Fam. Solanaceae) or a mixture of both species. It contains not less than 0.4% of the alkaloids of Belladonna Root, calculated as hyoscyamine.

Synonyms and Regional Names: Same as those of Belladonna Herb.

Morphology: Form – simple or occasionally branched, sub-cylindrical, entire or

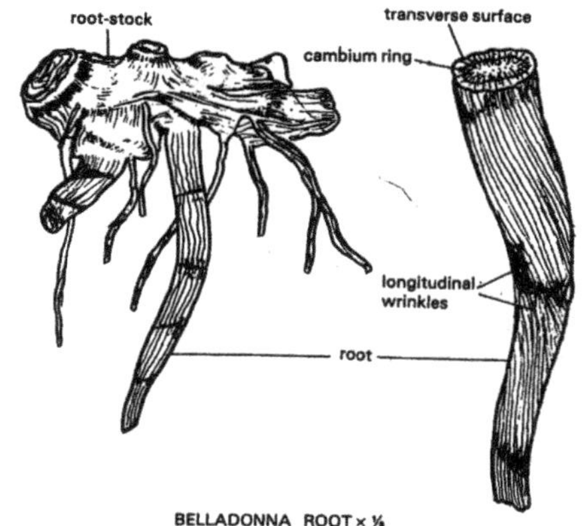

BELLADONNA ROOT × ⅓

longitudinally split; Colour – greyish brown; Size – 10.30 cm(l) and upto 4 cm(w) at the crown; Surface – longitudinally wrinkled; Fracture – short; Odour – not characteristic and Taste – bitter.

Active Constituents: Same as those of Belladonna Herb but only the alkaloidal percentage varies.

Therapeutical and Pharmaceutical Use: Same as those of Belladonna herb.

BENZOIN

Source: Benzoin is a balsamic resin obtained from *Styrax benzoin* Dryand or *S. paralleloneurus* Perkin, known in commerce as Sumatra Benzoin, or from *S. tonkinensis* (Pierre) Craib ex Hartwigh, known in commerce as Siam Benzoin (Fam. Styraceae). It contains not less than 25% of total balsamic acids, calculated with reference to dry alcohol soluble matter.

Synonyms and Regional Names: Gum benzoin Ben. Luban; Guj. Loban; Hin. Luban; Kan. Lobana; Mal. Sambrani; Mar. Luban; San. Sriloban; Tam. Shambirani; Tel. Sambrani.

Morphology: Form – appears as hard masses consisting of tears embedded in a translucent, reddish brown matrix. Size – varies; Surface – rough but smooth tears; Fracture – brittle; Odour – aromatic, balsamic and pleasant and Taste – slightly acrid.

Active Constituents:
SUMATRA BENZOIN
Balsamic acids – Cinnamic acid 20%
             – Benzoic acid 10%
Triterpenoid acids – Siaresinolic acid (19 hydroxy oleanolic acid)
                  – Sumaresinolic acid (6 hydroxy oleanolic acid)
Alcohol soluble extractive – not less than 70%
SIAM BENZOIN
Balsamic acids – Cinnmic acid in traces
             – Benzoic acid 10%
Coniferyl benzoate – 70%
Vanillin and some triterpenoid acids
Alcohol soluble extractive – not less than 90%

Therapeutical and Pharmaceutical Uses: 1. Expectorant 2. Antiseptic 3. Tincture is used in cosmetic solutions and as an inhalation aid in respiratory diseases.

Chemical Tests

1. Solubility: Insoluble in water but partially soluble in alcohol.
2. Benzoin when gradually heated, evolves white fumes of cinnamic and benzoic acids which on condensation form crystalline sublimate.
3. Siam benzoin gives a green colouration when its alcoholic extract is added to an alcoholic soln. of $FeCl_3$. Sumatra benzoin however, does not answer.
4. 2 g of coarse Sumatra benzoin is heated with 10 ml of 1% $KMnO_4$ soln. whereby bitter almond odour (oxidation of cinnamic acid) of benzaldehyde is produced. Siam benzoin because of its small quantity of cinnamic acid does not answer this test.

BITTER ALMOND

Source: Bitter almond is the seed of *Prunus amygdalus* Batsch. var. *amara* (Fam. Rosaceae).

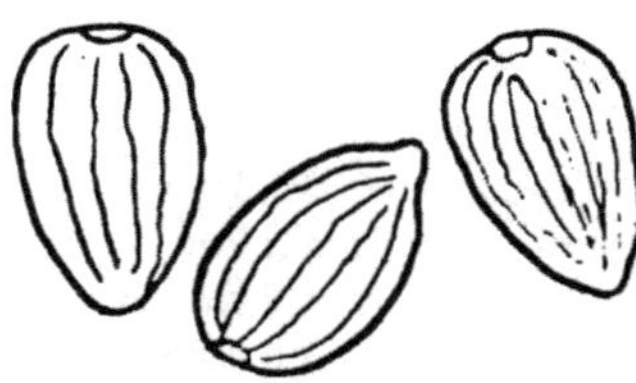

BITTER ALMOND SEEDS

Morphology: Size – 1.5 – 2 cm(l); Colour – Cinnamon brown; Form – rounded at one end and pointed at other; Taste – bitter.

Active Constituents: GLYCOSIDES – Cyanogenetic glycoside – Amygdalin (2.5 – 4%). FIXED OIL – (40 – 55%), PROTEINS, MUCILAGE, etc. VOLATILE OIL (Bitter almond oil) – Benzaldehyde (80%) – HCN (2 – 4%).

Therapeutical and Pharmaceutical Uses: 1. As an ingredient in cough remedies 2. As a vehicle for oily injections 3. As a flavouring agent.

BRAHMI

Source: Brahmi consists of fresh and dried leaves and stems of *Centella asiatica* Urban (Fam. Umbelliferae).

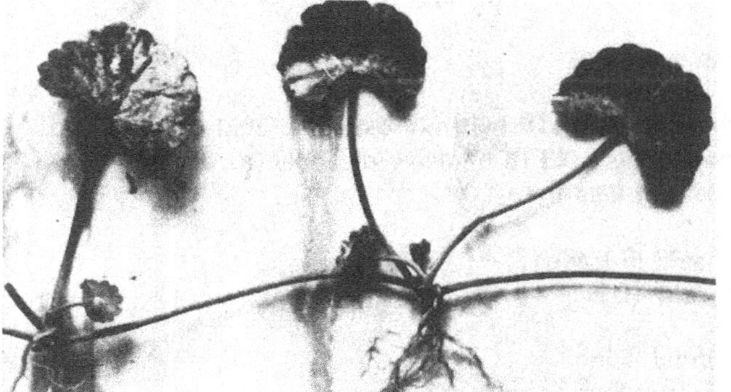

Synonyms and Regional Names

Hydrocotyle asiatica
Indian penny wort
Ben. Brahmamanduki, Tholkuri
Guj. Barmi
Hin. Brahmmanduki (also in Sanskrit)
Mar. Brahmi
Tam. Vallarei
Tel. Brahmi, Bokkudu

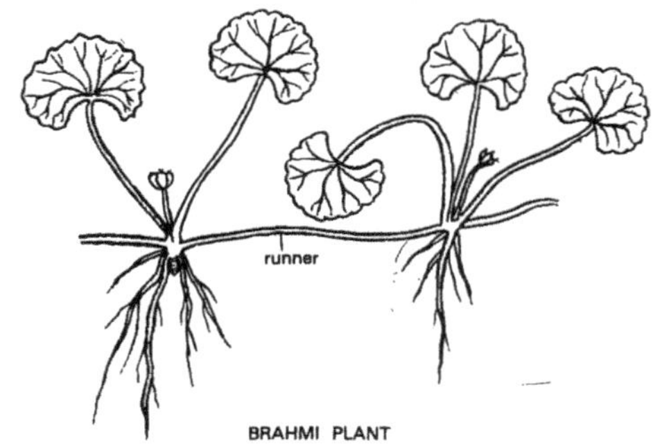

Morphology: Stems – long, prostrate, filiform, often reddish with long internodes rooting at the nodes; Leaves – 2 to 6 cm (d), reniform or orbicular-reniform, cordate, 1 to 3 from each node, entire, crenate, lobulate, glabrous and long petioled. Petiole – 7 to 15 cm (l), channelled, stipules short, adnate forming a sheathing base.

Active Constituents: GLYCOSIDES

– Saponin glycosides – Brahmoside, Brahminoside (0.16%) – Triterpene acids – Brahmic acid and isobrahmic acid – Brahmoside is a triglycoside of brahmic acid with rhamnose, glucose and arabinose as sugar components; whereas brahminoside is a tetraglycoside of brahmic acid. Another saponin glycoside Thankuniside yields on hydrolysis a triterpene acid, thankunic acid, glucose and rhamnose. Further two more saponins viz. Asiaticoside and oxyasiaticoside and the triterpene acids – asiatic acid, madecass acid and madasiatic acid.

Therapeutical and Pharmaceutical Uses; 1. Sedative 2. Antiprotozoal 3. In cases of epilepsy and other neurological conditions 4. Blood purifier, tonic, diuretic etc. 5. Anti-bacterial and to heal wounds. 6. Reported to heal peptic ulcer.

CAMPHOR

Source: Camphor is obtained from the wood of stems and roots of *Cinnamomum camphora* L. (Fam. Lauraceae).

Synonyms and Regional Names: Karpuram, Karpura.

Nature: Natural camphor is dextro-rotatory. It occurs as colourless to white crystalline powder or as transparent fibrous blocks; Odour – characteristic and pungent; Taste – aromatic, burning sensation followed by a cool feeling. At room temp. camphor volatilizes forming an incrustation on the walls of the container.

Chemical Constituents: TERPENOIDS

– Bicyclic monoterpene and Ketone. Other biproducts obtained from the wood are borneol, terpineol, 1 – 8 cineole, pinene, phellandrene, eugenol and safrole.

Therapeutical and Pharmaceutical Uses

1. As a topical antipruritic (an agent that counteracts itching).
2. Internally as a mild antiseptic and carminative.
3. Commercially used in the manufacture of certain plastics, celluloid etc.

CANNABIS

Source: Cannabis consists of the dried flowering tops of the cultivated pistillate plants of *Cannabis sativa* L. (Fam. Cannabinaceae).

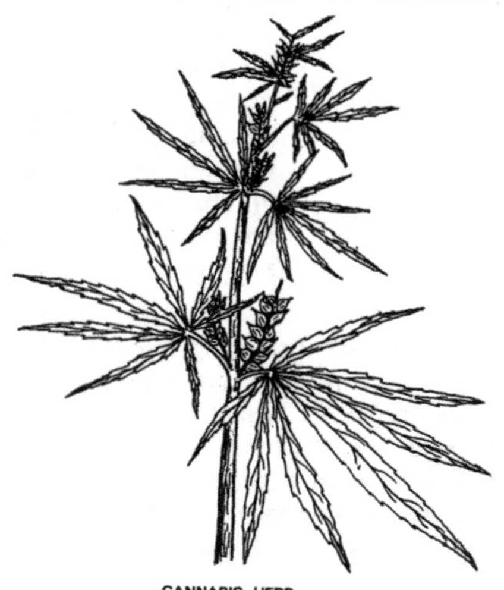

CANNABIS HERB

Synonyms and Regional Names
Indian Hemp, Hashish
Marihuana
Ben. Bhang
Guj. Ganja
Hin. Ganja, Bhang, Charas
Kan. Bhangi, Ganja
Mal. Kancavu, Kancha
Mar. Bhang, Ganja
San. Ganjika, Bhanga
Tam. Kanja
Tel. Ganjayi

Morphology: Form – compressed rough dusky green masses consisting of the branched upper part of the stem bearing leaves and pistillate flowers of fruits matted together by resinous secretion. Upper leaves simple, alternate; lower leaves opposite and digitate consisting of 5 – 7 linear-lanceolate leaflets. Fruit – one seeded, supported by an ovate-lanceolate bract. Odour – strong and characteristic (narcotic). Taste – acrid and pungent.

Active Constituents
RESINS (2.5% – 15%) — Tetrahydro cannabinol (THC)
Cannabidiolic acid (CBDA)

Therapeutical and Pharmaceutical Uses

1. Sedative (calms down excitement)
2. Analgesic (pain killer)
3. Hypnotic (induces sleep)
4. Psychotropic (exerting an effect upon the mind)
5. Antibacterial agent.

CANTHARIDES

Source: Cantharides consists of dried beetles – *Cantharis vesicatoria* L. (Fam. Meloidae).

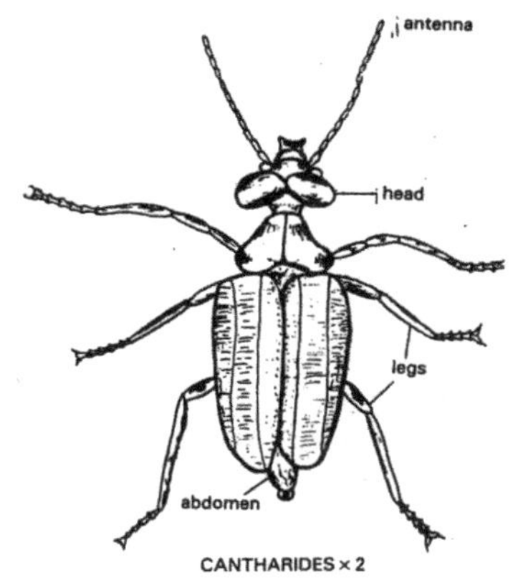

Synonyms and Regional Names
Spanish flies,
Russian flies
or Blistering flies.

Active Constituents: LACTONE –
Containing natural products – cantha-
ridin (0.6 to 1%), a lactone or an
anhydride of cantharidic acid –
–FAT (12%).

Therapeutical and Pharmaceutical Uses

1. An irritant, vesicant (an agent that produces blisters) and rubefacient (reddening of the skin).
2. Used against certain types of warts.
3. In hair tonics and Pomades.

CAPSICUM

Source: Capsicum consists of the dried ripe fruit of *Capsicum frutescens* L. or of C. *annuum* L. (Fam. Solanaceae). It contains not less than 12% of non-volatile ether extractives.

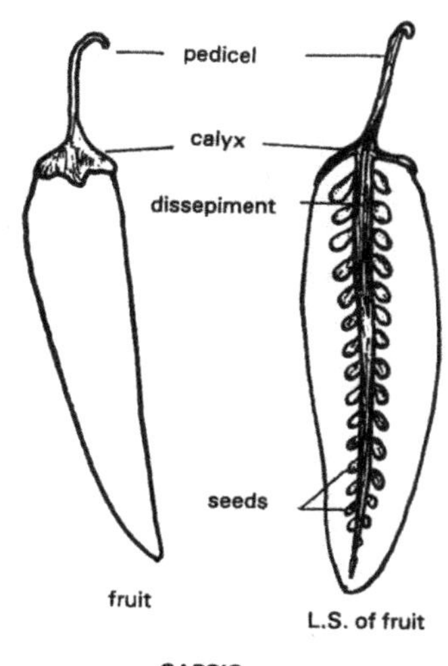

Synonyms and Regional Names: Chilli, Red pepper, Spanish pepper; Ben. Lal mirchi; Guj. Marchan; Hin. Lal-mircha; Kan. Mensinkay; Mal. Mulagu; Mar. Lal-mirchi; San. Marichiphalam; Tam. Pachemolaga; Tel. Mirpakayalu.

Morphology: Form – oblong conical, obtuse and 2-celled; Colour – dull orange red to brownish red; Size – 12 – 25 mm(l) and upto 7 mm maximum(w), attached to 5 toothed inferior calyx and a straight slender pedicel; Pericarp – somewhat shrivelled, glabrous and leathery containing about 10 – 20 brownish yellow, flat, subreniform seeds; Seeds – 3 – 4 mm(l), loose or attached to a thin reddish dissepiment; Odour – characteristic; Taste – pungent.

Active Constituents: PUNGENT PHENOLIC COMPOUNDS
— Capsaicinoids, a mixture of 5 isomeric acid amides – Capsaicin (70%) – Homocapsaicin – Dihydrocapsaicin – Homodihydrocapsaicin – Nordihydrocapsaicin.

CAROTENOIDS (0.12 – 0.35%)
ASCORBIC ACID (0.1 – 0.5%)
FIXED OIL
FLAVONOIDS

Therapeutical and Pharmaceutical Uses: 1. Carminative 2. Nerve stimulant 3. Increases the capillarity of the blood vessels 4. Source of Vitamin C 5. In galenic to treat cases of 'Rheuma arthritis' (rheumatism of joints).

CARAWAY

Source: Caraway consists of the dried ripe fruits of *Carum carvi* L. (Fam. Umbelliferae). It contains not less than 3.5% of volatile oil.

Synonyms and Regional Names: Caraway seed; Ben. Jira; Guj. Shahjiru; Hin. Shiajira, Zira, Vilaythi Zira; Kan. Jirige; Mal. Jirigam; Shahjira; San. Seeshavi; Tam. Shimaishembu; Tel. Shimaisapu.

Morphology: Type of Fruit – Cremocarp; Form – fruits elongated, slightly curved tapering on either sides, separate mericarps and detached from the pedicel; Size – 7 mm(l) and 2 mm(b). Colour – brown to greenish brown; Surface – glabrous with five primary ridges, thin pericarp and oily endosperm; Odour and Taste – aromatic and characteristic.

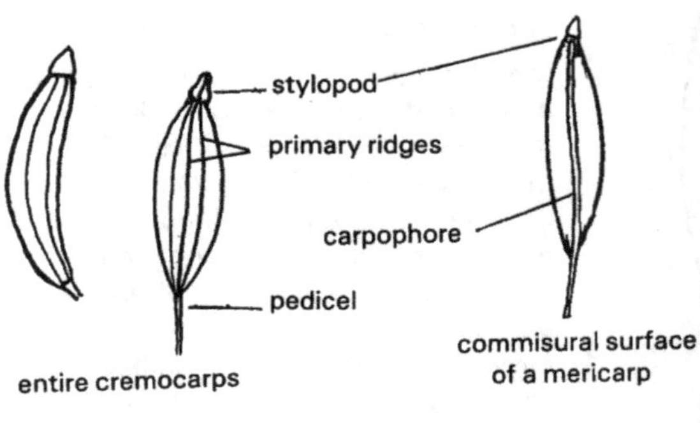

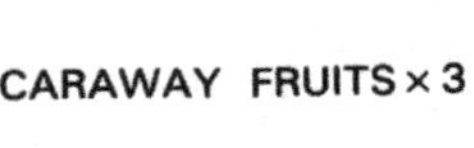

CARAWAY FRUITS × 3

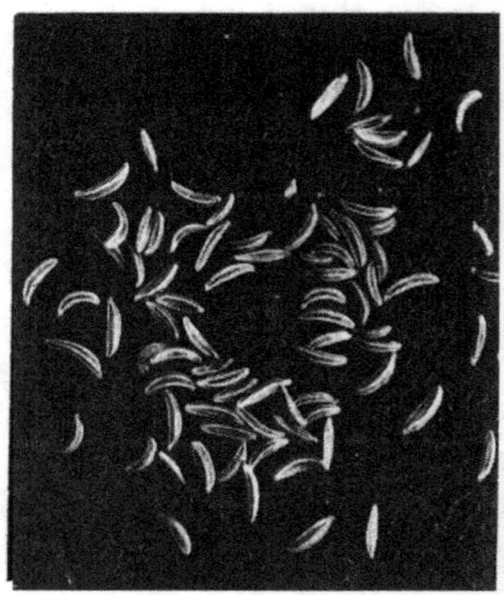

Active Constituents: VOLATILE OIL (3 – 7%) – d-Carvone (50 – 63%)
D-Limonene (30%), Carveol, Dihydrocarvone, Geraniol etc.
FATTY OIL (18 – 23%)
PROTEIN (21 – 23%)

Therapeutical and Pharmaceutical Uses

1. Spasmolytic (an agent which has the property to arrest sudden violent and involuntary muscular contraction).
2. Carminative (relieves the excessive collection of gas in the stomach).
3. As a spice.

Substitutes and Adulterants: Cumin fruits and some species of *Carum* are used as Jira in different parts of India. Cumin fruits are obtained from *Cuminum cyminum* (Umbelliferae). The volatile oil mainly contains cumin aldehyde and no carvone. Commercial samples contain both entire cremocarps and separate mericarps. While official caraway is curved, cumin fruits are ellipsoidal. Besides the 5 straight primary ridges, 4 secondary ridges occur over the vittae. Also characteristic are the bristles or short hairs found on the outer surface.

Fruits of *Carum bulbocastanum* appear as small, separate mericarps, oblong, semiterete and dark brown in colour and hence the name 'kala-jira'. While the vittae in *C. carvi* are all of the same size, in *C. bulbocastanum* two ventral vittae are smaller than dorsal vittae. Carvone is totally absent.

C. gracile is another commonly found substitute. Fruits are smaller in size and dorsally compressed with collapsed endocarp cells.

Finally it should be said that most of the commercial samples consist of a mixture of two or more fruits of different botanical source.

The following are the common adulterants:

1. Exhausted caraway. Here the essential oil of the drug is fully or partly withdrawn. However, based on organoleptic tests like colour, shape or form and odour, one can easily detect the exhausted drug which will be darker in colour, shrunken in nature and will have no characteristic aroma.
2. Excess of smaller stems and umbel rays. These in excess are usually admixed and this results in more of sclerenchymatous tissues and crude fibre.
3. Indian Dill consists of the fruits of *Anethum sowa*. The volatile oil of Indian Dill consists of more of Dill apiole and less of carvone. Reticulate parenchyma is another characteristic feature.

CARDAMOM

Source: Cardamom consists of the dried, nearly ripe fruit of *Elettaria cardamomum* Maton var. *minuscula* Burkill (Fam. Zingiberaceae), the seeds of which contain not less than 4% of volatile oil.

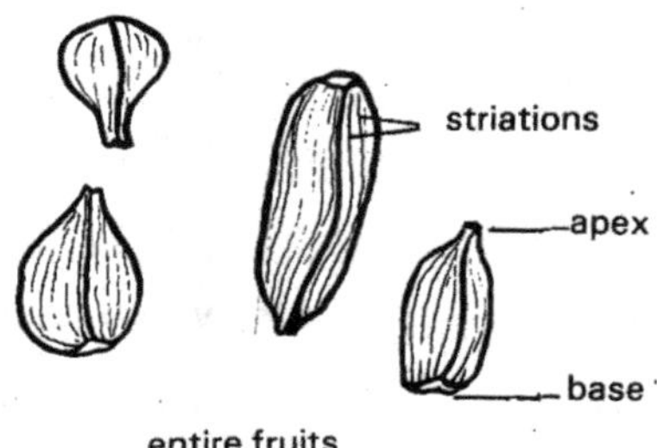

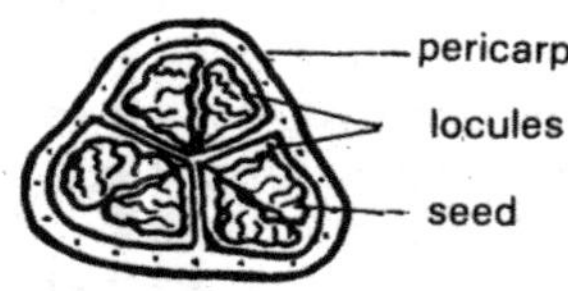

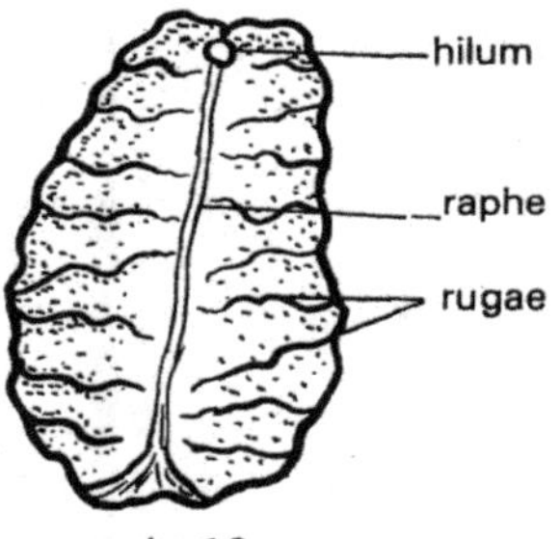

CARDAMOM

Synonyms and Regional Names: Cardamom, Lesser Cardamom; Ben. Elachi; Guj. Elachi; Hjn. Choti-ilaychi; Kan. Yalakki; Mal. Yelam; Mar. Veldoda; San. Ela; Tam. Elakkai; Tel. Elakayi.

Morphology: FRUIT: Condition – dry; Type – trilocular capsule; Size – varies from 1 to 2 cm; Shape – Ovoid or oblong; Apex – slightly pointed and beak like; Base – rounded and shows the remains of a stalk; Surface – smooth or with thin longitudinal striations; Colour – pale buff to pale greenish buff.

T.S. OF FRUIT: Shows 3 locules with axile placentation. There are 2 rows of seeds in each locule. Each seed is surrounded by a thin whitish papery layer called aril.

SEEDS: Size – upto 4 mm(l) and 3 mm (b); Shape – irregularly angular; Colour – dark brown or reddish brown; Surface – on one side there is a longitudinal groove which indicates the position of raphe. The hilum is situated in a depression at the narrower end. The seeds are transversely rugose with 6 – 8 rugae in the length of seed; Odour and Taste – aromatic.

Active Constituents

VOLATILE OIL – (3.5 – 7% in fruits and 8 – 9% in seeds) 1, 8-cineole (50%) L-Terpineol, Terpenylacetate, Limonene, Borneol.
STARCH (22 – 40%) and FATTY OIL.

Therapeutical and Pharmaceutical Uses

1. Carminative (relieves the excessive collection of gas in the stomach).
2. Flavouring agent.

Substitutes and Adulterants: *Elettaria cardamomum* var. *major* also called Long Wild Native Cardamom grows wild in Sri Lanka. The fruits are twice as big as official cardamom, dark brown in colour with coarse striations. The oil is less aromatic and has different composition. Though a good number of *Amomum* species are used from time to time in place of Cardamom, two species deserve mention here. Bengal

Cardamom (*A. aromaticum*) – Fruits are narrowly obovate with a number of narrow longitudinal membranous wings. Seeds without rugae and aromatic. Inspite of the high percentage of cineole, the characteristic odour of cardamom is lacking. Nepal or greater Cardamom (*A. subulatum*) – Fruits are as big as nutmeg. globose, dark reddish brown in colour, seeds are held together by a viscid sugary pulp and contains a good percentage of cineole.

CASCARA

Source: Cascara sagrada is the dried bark of *Rhamnus purshiana* DC. (Fam. Rhamnaceae) collected at least one year before being used.

Synonyms and Regional Names: American Frangula, Sacred bark, Chittem bark.

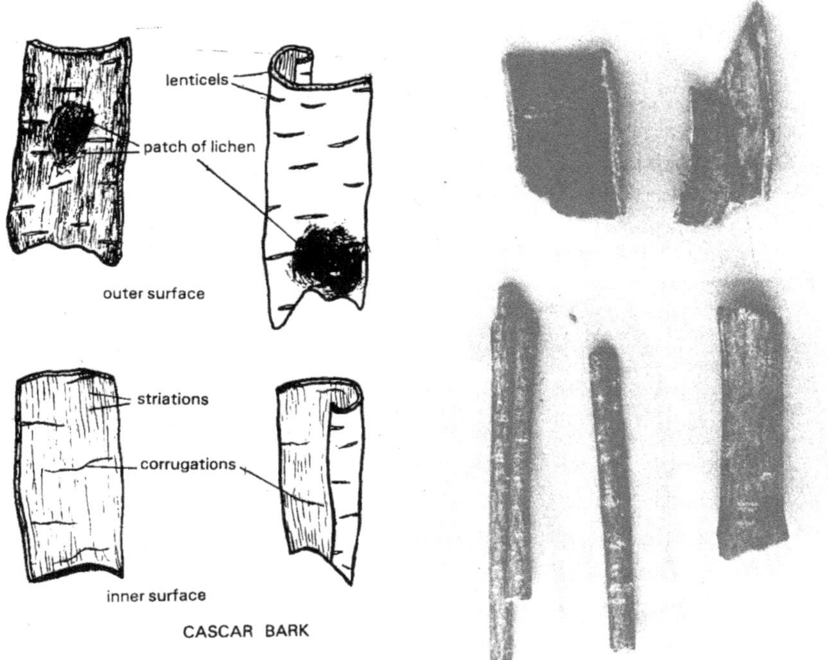

Morphology: Colour – dark, purple brown on the outerside and pale yellowish brown to black on the inner side; Shape – flat pieces, single quills and channelled also; Size – 5 to 20 cm(l), 1 to 4 mm(t) and upto 2 cm(w); Outer Surface – smooth with transversely elongated lenticels: Inner surface – definite fine longitudinal striations and faint transverse corrugations; Fracture – short and granular (outside) and fibrous in the phloem region; Odour – faint and Taste – persistently bitter and nauseous.

Active Constituents: GLYCOSIDES – Anthracene glycosides (8%)

1. C – glycosides (80 – 90%) comprising
   a) Cascarosides A and B (Stereo isomers of Barbaloin-O-β-d-glucoside)
   b) Cascarosides C and D (Stereo isomers of Chrysaloin-8-O-β-d-glucoside)
   c) Barbaloin
   d) Chrysaloin.
2. O-glycoside (10 – 20%) – Frangula emodin oxanthrone glucoside.
3. Homodianthrones of emodin, aloe-emodin and chrysophanol.
4. Heterodianthrones like palmidin A, B and C.
5. Emodin, Aloe-emodin and chrysophanol as free aglycones.

Therapeutical and Pharmaceutical Uses: Cathartic (promoting active movement of bowels). It·rectifies the habitual constipation where it not only acts as a laxative but restores natural tone to the colon.

Chemical Test: Constituents of Cascara answer Borntrager's test. For details see Senna.

CASSIA

Source: Cassia consists of the dried stem bark of *Cinnamomum cassia* Blume (Fam. Lauraceae). It contains not less than 1.0% v/w volatile oil.

Synonym and Regional Name: Chinese Cinnamon.

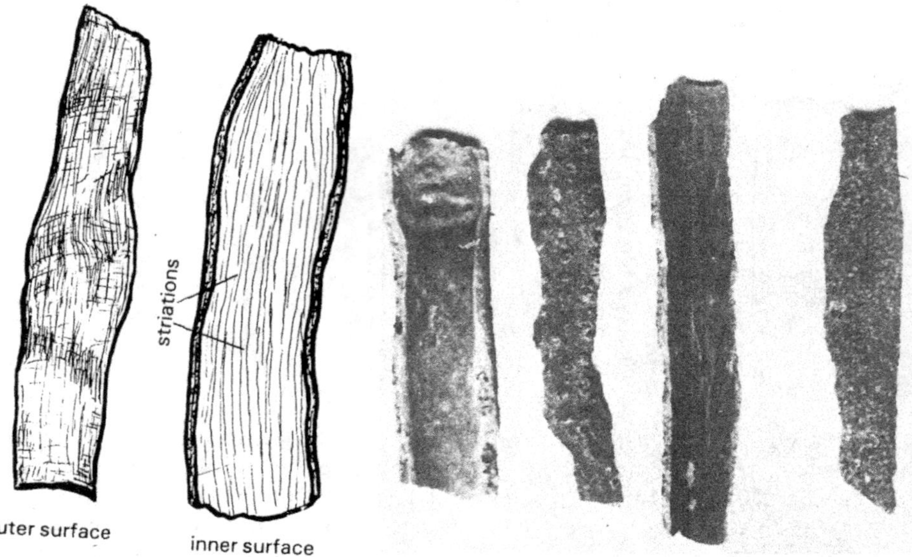

CASSIA BARK

Morphology: Condition – dry, Shape – channelled, single quills; Size – length upto 40 cm; width 1 to 2 cm, thickness 1 to 5 mm; Ex. surface – darker than Cinnamon and shows cork patches due to careless planning; In-surface – brownish with fine striations; Odour and Taste – coarser than that of Cinnamon and more astringent.

Active Constituents: VOLATILE OIL (1 – 2%) – Cinnamic aldehyde (75 – 90%) – Terpene aldehyde and esters. Eugenol which is present in Cinnamon is totally absent here.

Therapeutical and Pharmaceutical Uses

1. Flavouring agent.
2. As a mild astringent.
3. Powerful germicide (oil).

Chemical Test: Refer Cinnamon.

Note: Cassia bark is a cheap substituent to Cinnamon bark (page 42).

CASTOR OIL

Source: Castor Oil is the fixed oil obtained by cold expression from the seeds of *Ricinus communis* L. (Fam. Euphorbiaceae).

Synonyms and Regional Names: Ben. Bherenda, Guj. Diveli, Hin. Erand, Kan. Haralenne, Mal. Amanakku, Mar. Erand, San. Erendi, Tam. Amanakku chedi Tel. Amudamu.

Characters: Colour – colourless or pale yellow; Nature – viscid liquid; Odour – faint; Taste – acrid and nauseating; Solubility – soluble in alcohol in all proportions.

Active Constituents: LIPIDS – Fixed Oils (45 to 55%)
– a mixture of triglycerides
– Triricinolein (75%) which on hydrolysis yields Ricinoleic acid responsible for the cathartic effect.

Therapeutical and Pharmaceutical Uses

1. Cathartic (increases the movement of the bowels)
2. In soap industry. 3. As a lubricant.

Chemical Test:

1. When mixed with equal volume of dehydrated alcohol, the soln. remains clear.
2. When treated with half of its volume petroleum ether (50 – 60°) it mixes completely but with twice its volume it becomes turbid and partly soluble.

CATECHU (Black)

Source: Black Catechu consists of the dried aqueous extract prepared from the heart wood of *Acacia catechu* Willd. and *A. chundra* Willd. (Fam. Leguminosae).

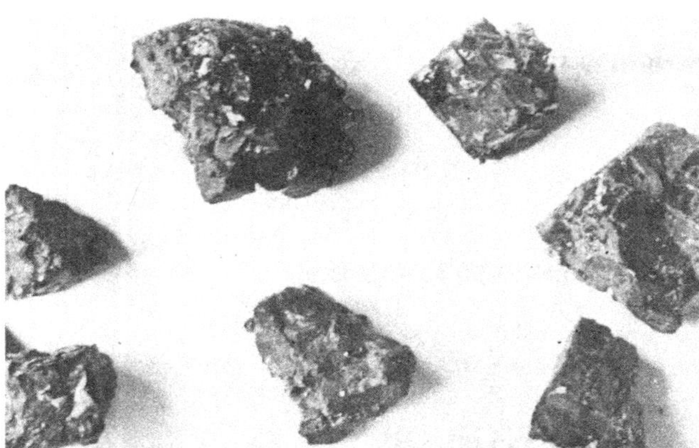

Synonyms and Regional Names
Cutch tree
Ben.Khaer
Guj. Khato
Hin. Khair, Kattha
Kan. Cachu
Mal. Karinali,
    Khadiram
Mar. Khair
San.Khadira
Tam. Karunkali
Tel. Chandra

Morphology: Colour – black or dark brown; Form – irregular masses or cubes; Surface – rough, dull or slightly glossy and porous; Fracture – very brittle breaking into powdery mass; Odour – none; Taste – bitter to start with, turns sweet and finally astringent.

Active Constituents

TANNINS – Catechins (2 – 12%), Catechutannic acid (25 – 60%) a condensation product of Acacatechin.

FLAVONOIDS – Quercetin and its derivatives.

Therapeutical and Pharmaceutical Uses: 1. Astringent (arrests discharges or secretions).   2. Cooling and digestive.   3. Used in relaxed conditions of throat, mouth and gums.

Chemical Tests
1. Completely soluble in hot water and alcohol.
2. Test for Tannin: A 10% filtered aqueous soln. of the drug gives a dark green colour with a 5% solutions of $FeCl_3$. Colour changes to purple on making the soln. slightly alkaline with a soln. of NaOH.
3. To a few drops of fresh aqueous extract, 10 ml of lime water is added whereby a brown colouration is produced which on standing for a couple of minutes gives red precipitate.
4. With Vanillin hydrochloric (conc.) acid, black catechu (dry powder) shows pink or red colour due to the production of phloroglucinol.

CATECHU (Pale)

Source: Pale catechu or Gambier consists of the dried aqueous extract prepared from the leaves and shoots of *Uncaria gambier* Hunt. (Fam. Rubiaceae)

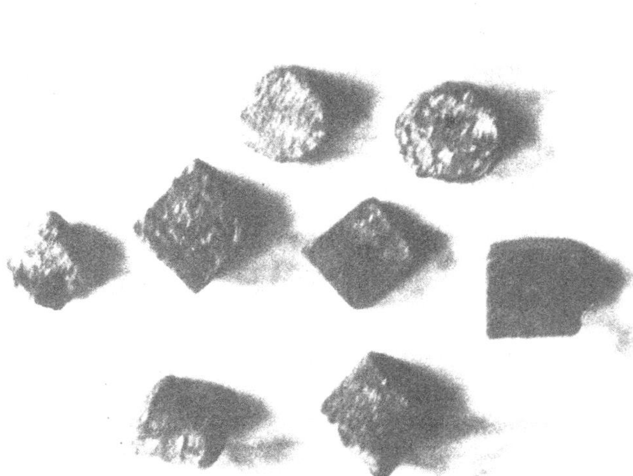

Synonyms and Regional Names
Gambier, Gambir
Guj. Katho
Hin. Kattha, Catechu

Morphology
Colour — dull greyish brown to dark reddish brown externally and pale brown internally;
Form: smaller cubes;
Surface — dull,
Fracture — Brittle;
Odour, Taste and Solubility — similar to black catechu.

Active Constituents: TANNINS (Condensed tannins) — Catechins (7 to 33%) Catechu tannic acid (22 to 50%)
FLAVONOIDS — Quercetin and a fluorescent substance — Gambir fluorescin.

Therapeutical and Pharmaceutical Uses: 1. Astringent 2. Used in cases of diarrhoea 3. Used in dye and tanning industries.

Chemical Tests: Though pale catechu answers the tests of black catechu as well, it differs in answering positively two other tests based on the presence of (a) Gambir fluorescin and (b) Chlorophyll obtained from leaves and shoots of the plant.
1. Warm 0.3 g of powdered catechu in 2 ml alcohol. Filter. Add 2 ml of NaOH soln. and 2 ml of light petroleum to the filtrate. Shake and allow it to stand. On standing, two layers separate out and the petroleum layer emits a green fluorescence.
2. 1 g of the drug is extracted with 5 ml of Chloroform. On filtering a green colour can be seen in the filtrate.

CHAULMOOGRA OIL

Source: Chaulmoogra Oil is the fatty oil obtained by cold expression from the fresh ripe seeds of *Hydnocarpus kurzii*(King) Warb. (Farm. Flacourtiaceae) or other species of *Hydnocarpus*.

Synonym and Regional Name: Chaulmoogra tel.

Nature: Colour – yellow to brownish yellow; state – below 25° a white soft solid; Odour – characteristic, somewhat similar to that of rancid butter; Taste – acrid.

Active Constituents: Mixture of Glycerides
FATTY ACIDS – Hydnocarpic acid (35.3%) – Chaulmoogric acid (22.7%) – Gorlic acid (22.8%) – Oleic acid (14.8%) – Palmitic acid (4%).

Therapeutical and Pharmaceutical Uses: In the treatment of leprosy and tuberculosis.

CHENOPODIUM OIL

Source: Chenopodium Oil is a volatile oil obtained by steam distillation from the fresh flowering and fruiting plants (excluding root) of *Chenopodium ambrosioides* L.var. *anthelminticum.* A. Gray (Fam. Chenopodiaceae).

Synonyms: Oil of Mexican tea, Oil of American wormseed.

Nature: Colour – Pale yellow to orange yellow; Odour – characteristic, penetrating, camphoraceous; Taste – burning bitter.

Chemical Nature: ESSENTIAL OIL (1 – 2%) – Peroxide – Ascaridol (65 – 70%), an unsaturated terpene peroxide (Ascaridol is liable to explode when heated), p-cymol, limonene, camphor, α terpineol, pinene.

Therapeutical and Pharmaceutical Uses

1. As an anthelminticum especially for round and hookworms.
2. In combination also for intestinal infections.

Note: Oil should be used with great care.

CHIRATA

Source: Chirata is the plant *Swertia chirata* Buch. Ham. (Fam. Gentianaceae) collected when in flower and dried. Chirata contains not less than 1.3% of the bitter principle.

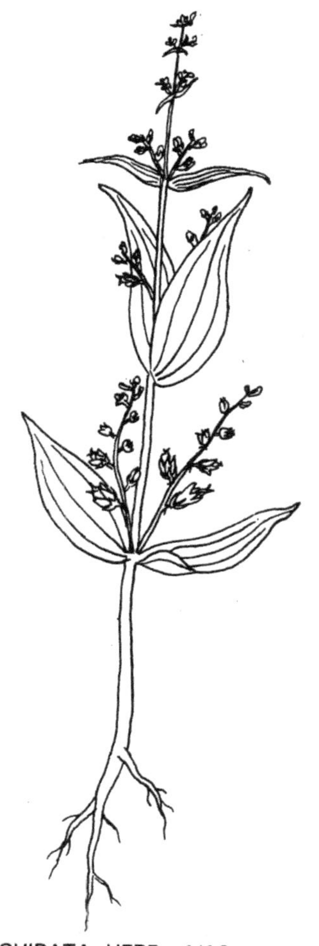

CHIRATA HERB × 1/10

Synonyms and Regional Names: Indian Gentian, Chiretta, Ben. Chireta; Guj. Charayatah; Hin. Chirayata; Kan. Kirata Kaddi; Mal. Kiriyattu; Mar. Charayatah; San. Kirata-tikta, Bhunimba; Tam. Nilavembu.

Morphology: Stem being the principal portion of the drug measures upto about 1 m(l); Colour – purplish brown; Shape – slightly winged and much branched above, branches slender; opposite, decussate; Leaves – opposite, ovate or lanceolate, glabrous and entire; Flowers – small and numerous, panicled; Fruits – superior, bicarpellary unilocular containing numerous seeds; Odour – none and Taste – extremely bitter.

Active Constituents
BITTER PRINCIPLES (1.4 – 1.5%)
— Ophelic acid – Chiratin
— Amarogentin.

Therapeutical and Pharmaceutical Uses
1. Bitter tonic
2. Stomachic (a gastric stimulant)
3. Febrifuge (an agent to reduce the fever).

CHRYSAROBIN

Source: Chrysarobin is a mixture of neutral principles obtained from Goa powder, a substance deposited in the trunks of *Andira araroba* Aguiar (Fam. Leguminosae).

Note: (Powder irritates mucous membrane).

Synonyms: Goa Powder, Araroba.

Active Constituents: GLYCOSIDES – Anthracene derivatives, chrysophanol anthranol, Chrysophanol anthrone (30 – 40%) and other anthraquinone derivatives.

Therapeutical and Pharmaceutical Use: As an antiseptic in skin infections and as well as a parasiticide.

Chemical Tests: 1. Answers tests for anthracene derivatives (of aloes, senna etc.). 2. Chrysarobin 2mg + Fuming nitric acid (2 drops)→ Red brown colour. On addition of a few drops of dil. ammonia solution the colour changes to violet red. 3. A dark brownish red colour is produced on dissolving 0.1 g of chrysarobin in 10 ml of hot soln. of NaOH. 4. On dissolving 0.1 g of chrysarobin in H_2SO_4 a deep red soln. is produced. Pour the soln. in water, chrysarobin separates.

CINCHONA

Source: Cinchona is the dried bark of cultivated trees of *Cinchona calisaya* Wedd., *C. ledgeriana* Moens, *C. officinalis* L, *C. succirubra* Pav. ex-Klotzsch or of hybrids of either of the last two species with either of the first two (Fam. Rubiaceae). It contains not less than 6% of total alkaloids of Cinchona.

Synonyms
Cinchona bark, Jesuit's bark, Peruvian bark

Morphology
Condition – dry
Shape – flat, channelled, single quill or double quill
Size – varies; Outer surface – yellowish brown or reddish brown or greyish. Surface is rough

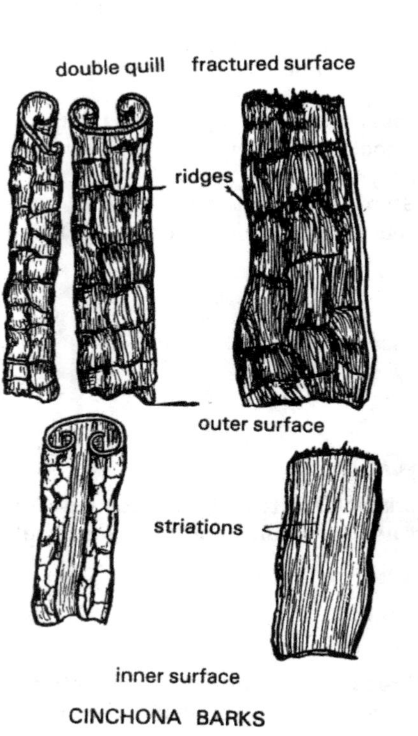

CINCHONA BARKS

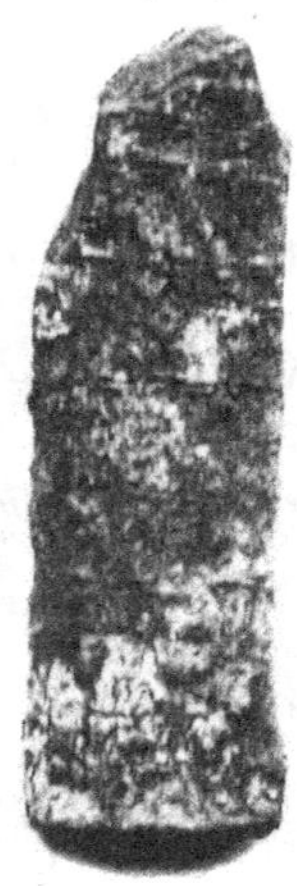
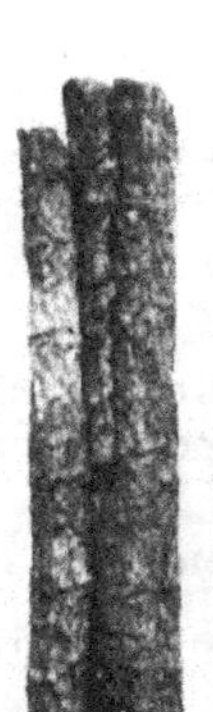
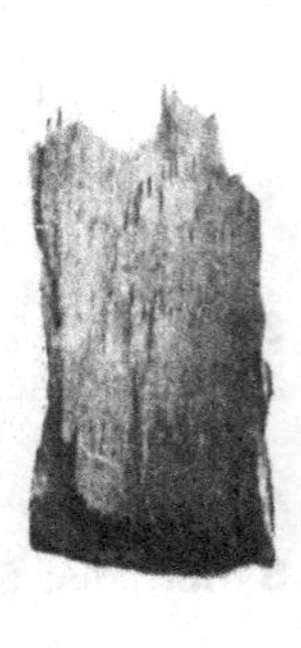

due to longitudinal and transverse ridges, fissures and wrinkles. At times greyish patches of lichens may be seen; Inner surface: dark reddish brown or pale yellowish brown with longitudinal striations; Fracture — short in the outer region and fibrous in the phloem region; Taste — bitter and astringent; Odour — characteristic.

Microscopy (Transverse Section)

T. S. Shows a well developed periderm, a wide cortex and a large secondary phloem.

PERIDERM

Cork consists of several layers of radially arranged rows of thin walled cells with dark brown contents. The cork cells are impregnated with suberin.

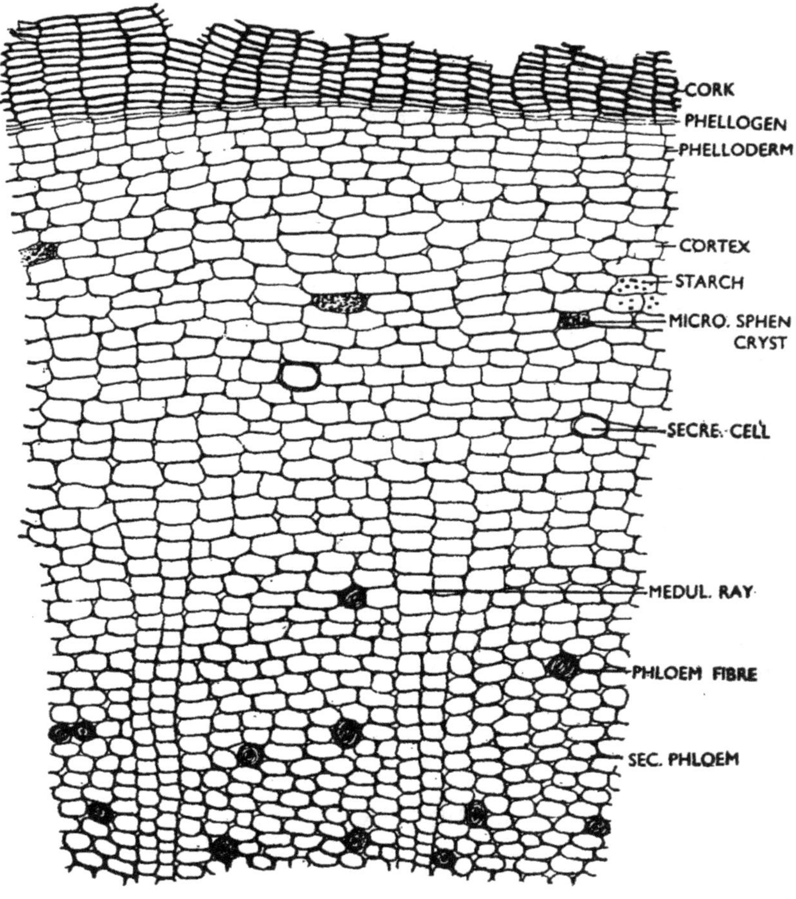

Cinchona Bark. T. S. (X 100)

Phellogen 2 to 3 layers of thin walled rectangular cells without any cellular contents.

Phelloderm 6 to 8 layers of thin walled rectangular cells without any cellular contents. Like cork, they are arranged at times in radial rows.

Cortex several layers of thin walled and tangentially elongated cells containing yellowish brown matter. Some of the cortical cells are filled with microsphenoidal crystals of calcium oxalate and the rest with minute starch grains. Besides, isolated secretion cells (latex ducts) are also found in the cortical parenchyma.

SECONDARY PHLOEM consists of phloem parenchyma, phloem fibres and medullary rays.

Phloem fibres, characteristic of Cinchona bark occur intermingled with phloem parenchyma and in between medullary rays. Fibres numerous, mostly isolated, at times in groups of 2 or 3, rounded to oval, in various sizes, yellow in colour, thick walled, strongly lignified with a small lumen and stratifications.

MEDULLARY RAYS traverse radially the phloem parenchyma; 1 – 3 cells wide, extend upto cortex, cells radially elongated and contain starch grains.

Active Constituents: ALKALOIDS (6 – 7%) – Quinoline alkaloids. Quinine (50 – 60%), Quinidine, Cinchonine, Cinchonidine.
QUINOVIN – a bitter glycoside also responsible for the bitter taste, yields on hydrolysis quinovaic acid and quinovose, a sugar derivative.
TANNINS – Phlobatannins.

Therapeutical and Pharmaceutical Uses: 1. In the treatment of malarial fever. 2. In the preparation of tonic water. 3. Quinidine is also used as a cardiac depressant. It is categorized as anti-arrhythmic and anti-fibrillatory drug.

Chemical Tests: Thalleioquin Test: Residue of bark extract + 1 drop of dil. H_2SO_4 + 1 ml H_2O. To this mixture bromine water is added dropwise till a permanent yellow tinge is obtained and then on addition of 1 ml dil. ammonia soln. emerald green colour is obtained indicating the presence of quinoline alkaloids.

Substitutes: Cuprea bark (*Remijia pedunculata* and *R. purdiena*). Family Rubiaceae. The barks are copper red in colour and hard. Fracture – granular and splintery. Bark contains quinine and quinidine to the tune of 2 – 3%. The distinguishing histological character is the presence of stone cells which is totally absent in Cinchona.

Adulterants: In view of the very low percentage of the alkaloids in *C. calisaya* and *C. succirubra* these are sometimes considered as adulterants of *C. ledgeriana*

CINNAMON

Source: Cinnamon is the dried inner bark of the shoots of coppiced tree of *Cinnamomum zeylanicum* Blume. (Fam. Lauraceae) and is known in commerce as Ceylon Cinnamon. It contains not less than 1.0% v/w of volatile oil.

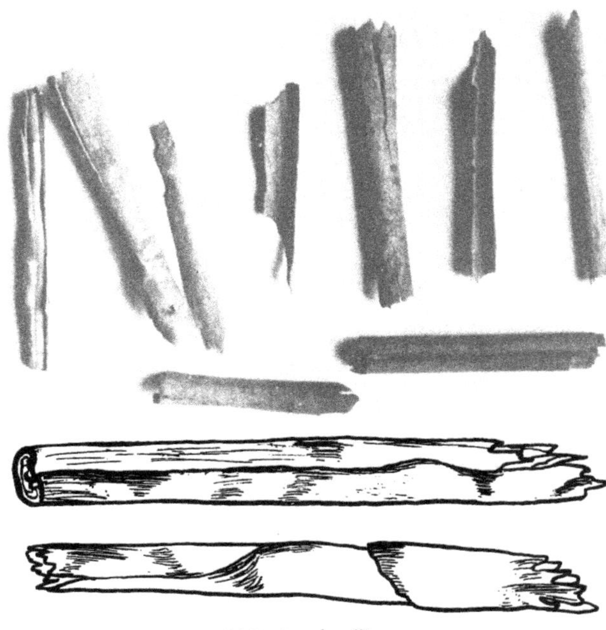

Synonyms and Regional Names
Ceylon cinnamon
Ben. Dalchini
Guj. Ceylon Taj
Hin. Dalchini
Kan. Dalchini
    lavangapatte
Mal. Karuvappatta,
    lavangam
Mar. Dalchini
Tam. Lavangapattai
Tel. Lavangapatta

Morphology: Condition – dry; Shape – single, double or compound quills; Size – varying length, 6 – 10 mm in diameter, thickness not more than 0.5 mm; Ex. surface.– yellowish brown with shining wavy lines of pericyclic fibres; In. surface – darker, straignt striations; Fracture – short and splintery; Taste – warm, sweet and aromatic; Odour – fragrant.

Active Constituents: VOLATILE OIL (0.8 – 1.4%) – Cinnamic aldehyde (60 – 75%) Phenol (chiefly Eugenol, 4 – 10%) Hydrocarbons, Alcohols etc.

PHLOBATANNIN and MUCILAGE

Therapeutical and Pharmaceutical Uses: 1. Flavouring Agent 2. As a mild astringent 3. Powerful germicide (oil).

Chemical Test: When a drop of ferric chloride soln. is added to 5 ml alcohol containing one drop of cinnamon oil, a pale green colour is obtained because of the following reactions:

Cinnamic aldehyde + $FeCl_3 \rightarrow$ Brown colour. Eugenol (with phenolic OH group) + $FeCl_3 \rightarrow$ Blue; together gives an intermediate green colour.

Substitutes and Adulterants: Cassia bark (page 34) is often sold in place of Cinnamon which is of superior quality. However, based on the presence or absence of cork, length and breadth of phloem fibres, size of starch grains and the presence or absence of eugenol, one can easily distinguish the two.

CLOVE

Source: Clove is the dried flower bud of *Eugenia caryophyllus* (Spreng.) Sprague (*Syzygium aromaticum,* (L) Merill et. L.M. Perry) Fam. Myrtaceae . It contains not less than 15% of clove oil.

Synonyms and Regional Names: Clove,Ben. Lavang; Guj. Laving; Hin. Laung; Kan. Lavanga; Mal. Grambu; Mar. Lavang; San. Lavangaha; Tam. Lavangam; Tel. Lavangalu.

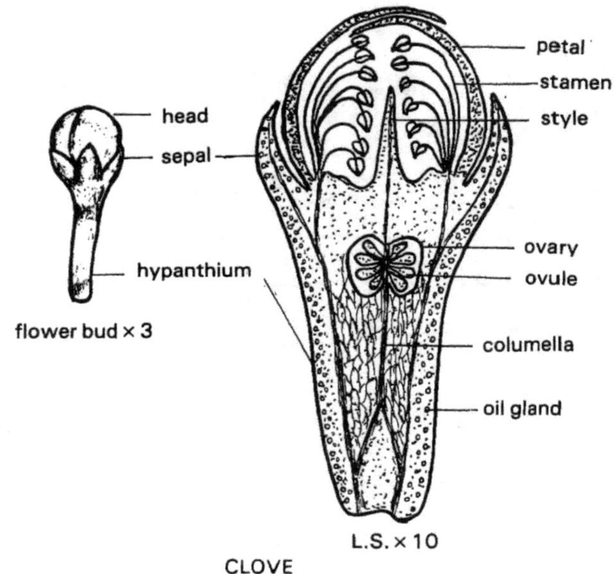

CLOVE

Morphology: Size – length varies from 12 to 17 mm; Type – actinomorphic, bisexual, epigynous. The flower bud has a spherical head and a sub-cylindrical hypanthium tapering at the lower end; Calyx – polysepalous, 4 hard and thick sepals with oil glands; Corolla – polypetalous, 4 petals imbricate, enclose the stamens and forms the head of the bud; Androecium – numerous stamens, free and introrse; Gynoecium – bilocular, inferior ovary with ovules (many) and placentation axile. Style-single and erect; Colour – dark brown; Odour – aromatic, strong; Taste – pungent, aromatic. The volatile oil is situated in the oil glands or ducts which are present in all parts of the flower bud.

Active Constituents: VOLATILE OIL (16 – 21%) – Phenol chiefly Eugenol (80 – 88%), Acetyl eugenol (10 – 15%),Humulen (5 – 12%), α and β – Caryophyllene TANNINS – (10 – 13%)

Therapeutical and Pharmaceutical Uses: 1. Antiseptic 2. Stimulant 3. Aromatic.

Substitutes and Adulterants: As per the official definition, clove bud should contain clove oil between 15 and 21% and not less. Sub-standard products will have obviously less than 15%. Over ripe buds and immature buds do not contain the prescribed percentage of oil. At times the oil is withdrawn intentionally and cloves free of oil is mixed with genuine drug or sold as such. The following are the usual adulterants.

1. *Exhausted clove:* Volatile oil is partly or completely removed. As a result buds appear darker in colour, shrunken in form and yield no oil even after pressing hard between the fingers.
2. *Clove stalks:* The stalks, which creep-in while collecting the buds, when present in excess are considered as adulterants. These stalks do not contain essential oil but only to the tune of 5%. It is easy to spot them out as they appear dark brown, angular, trichotomously branched, with nodes enlarged and with high percentage of crude fibre (13.6%). The crude fibre in official clove varies between 6 2 to 9.8%. If in powdered form, excess of clove stalk can be made out by the presence of calcium oxalate prisms and large thick walled stone cells which however are absent in official clove powder.
3. *Clove fruit (Mother clove or Anthophylli):* These also contain clove oil but only around 3 to 5% and hence considered as an adulterant. These cloves are distinctly longer (20 to 25 mm/10 – 17 mm), ovate and taper below. The single seed present in the fruit contains starch which is absent in clove bud. Using a simple microchemical test for starch, the adulterant can be detected.
4. *Blown clove:* Here mature clove flowers without corolla and stamens are also admixed. These eventually are very low in their oil content.

COCAINE

Source: Cocaine is an alkaloid obtained from the leaves of *Erythroxylon coca* Lamarck and its varieties (Fam. Erythroxylaceae) = *Erythroxylum coca*

Chemical Nature: ALKALOID – Tropane alkaloid. Cocaine is the methyl ester of benzoyl ecgonine which on hydrolysis yields ecgonine, benzoic acid and methyl alcohol.

Therapeutical and Pharmaceutical Uses: 1. Local anaesthetic 2. Cerebral stimulant 3. Narcotic.

COLCHICUM

Source: Colchicum corm and seed are dried corm and ripe seed of *Colchicum luteum* Baker (Fam. Liliaceae), respectively.

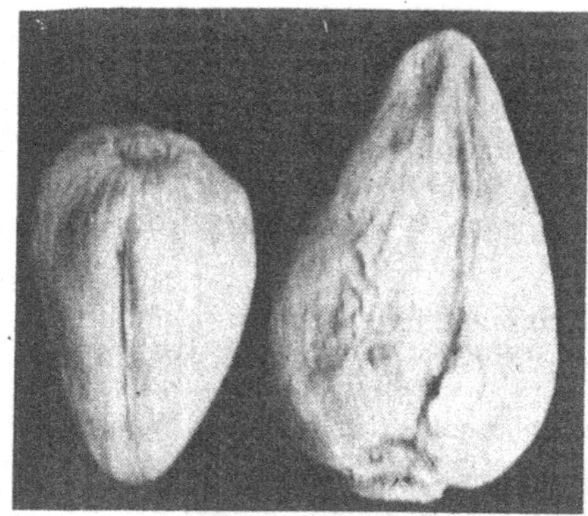

Colchicum Corms

Synonyms and Regional Names Indian colchicum, Meadow Saffron corm Hin. Hirantutiya, Surinjan San. Hiranyatutha

Morphology Corm: Form – conical rounded on one side flattened on the other with a groove in the middle running throughout the length of the corm; Colour – yellowish white; Surface – smooth; Fracture – short and mealy. Odourless and bitter taste. Seeds; Colour – light brown; Form – ovoid or irregularly globular; Size – 2-3 mm (d); Peculiarities – minutely pointed at the hilum

and with a distinct break approximately opposite to the hilum. Odourless and bitter taste.

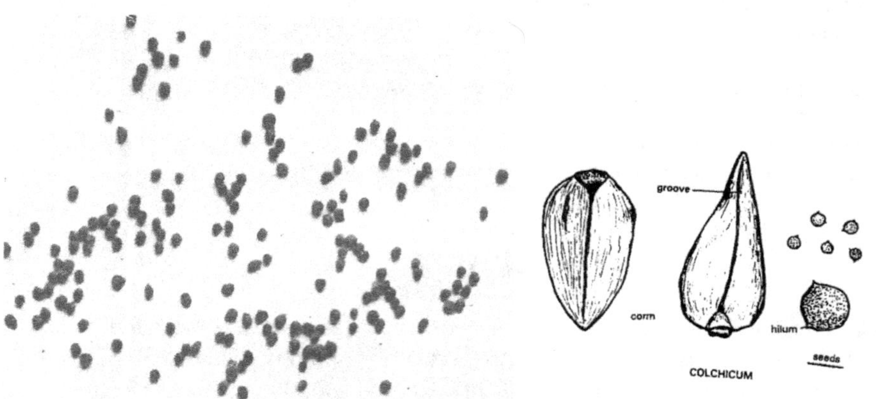

Colchicum Seeds

Active Constituents

ALKALOIDS — Colchicine type containing tropolone ring (0.5 to 1.0%)
     — Colchicine (0.8% in seeds and 0.6% in corms) – demecolcine.

Chemical Test: The alkaloid colchicine present both in the corm and seed yields an yellow colour with conc. HCl or 60 – 70% H_2SO_4.

Therapeutical and Pharmaceutical Uses

1. To relieve gout (inflammation of the joints)
2. Demecolcine is effectively used against epidermal cancer and myeloid leukaemia.
3. Colchicine is used to induce Polyploidy. (chromosomal multiplication).

COLOCYNTH

Source: Colocynth is the dried pulp of the unripe but full-grown fruit of *Citrullus colocynthis* L. Schrader (Fam. Cucurbitaceae).

Synonyms and Regional Names: Bitter apple, Ben. Indrayan; Guj. Indrak (Indra Varnu); Hin. Indrayan; Kan. Tumtikai; Mal. Peyikommutti; Mar. Indrayana, Kaduvrindava; San. Indravaruni; Tam. Pei-komatti; Tel. Verripuchchakaya

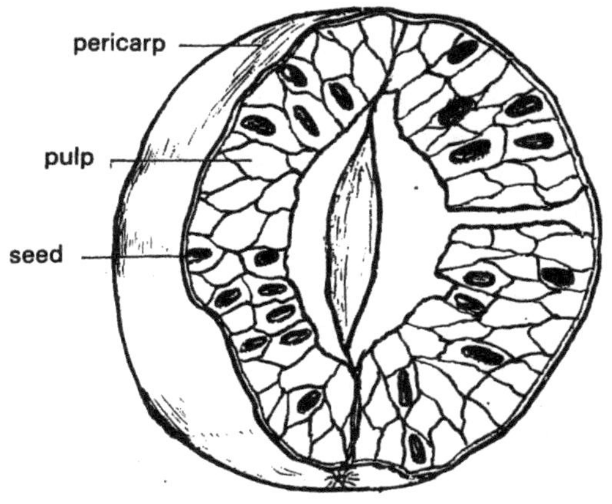

L.S. of fruit

COLOCYNTH

Morphology: Type of Fruit – berry; Shape – globular; Colour – unpeeled fruits have yellowish brown rind; Pericarp – hard and brittle; Pulp – white to pale yellowish and light in weight; Seeds – numerous, ovoid, flattened, pointed at one end with yellowish brown colour. The pulp has no odour but an intensely bitter taste.

Active Constituents: RESINS – triterpenoids – Cucurbitacins – Cucurbitacin E&I. (free and in glycoside form). PHYTOSTEROL GLYCOSIDES, BITTER PRINCIPLES.

Therapeutical and Pharmaceutical Use: Powerful cathartic (drastic purgative).

COLOPHONY

Source: Colophony is the solid residue obtained after distilling the oleo-resin from various species of *Pinus like P. longifolia, P. echinata, P. palustris and P. maritima* (Fam. Pinaceae).

Synonyms and Regional Names: Long needle pine; Ben. Saralagachha; Hin. Chir; San. Sarala; Tam. Simai Devadari; Tel. Sarala.

Morphology: Form – angular masses, glassy and irregular; Colour – pale or brownish yellow; Size – varies; Surface – smooth; Fracture – brittle; Odour and Taste – faintly terbinthinate. Solubility – being a resin, insoluble in water but soluble in alcohol, ether, benzene, glacial acetic acid and light petroleum.

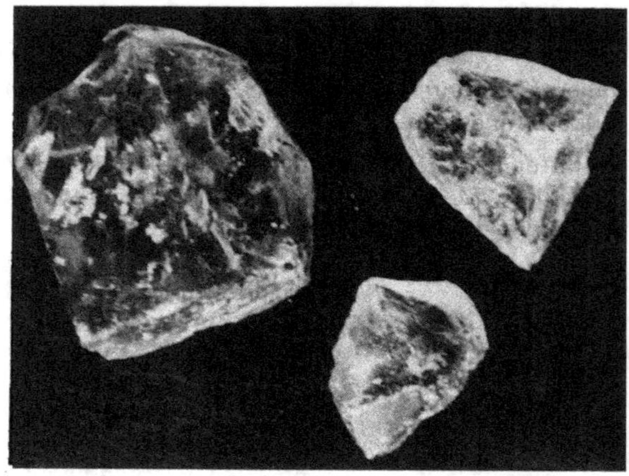

Active Constituents: RESIN ACIDS – Resin acid or diterpene acids like abietic acid (90%) – Neutral inert substance (Resenes), Ester of fatty acids.

Therapeutical and Pharmaceutical Uses: 1. In ointments and medicinal plasters. 2. Manufacturing of varnishes and disinfectant liquids.

Chemical Tests: 1. 0.1 g of powdered colophony is dissolved in 2 – 3 ml of acetic anhydride in a test tube and a drop of Con. H_2SO_4 is added whereby purple to violet colour is observed. 2. An alcoholic solution of colophony is acidic to litmus. 3. Colophony is dissolved in light petroleum and filtered. To the filtrate 2 to 3 times its volume, dil. copper acetate soln. is added whereby emerald green colour is seen in the petroleum layer (upper layer). (Fresh powder. Old powder is less soluble in light petroleum).

CORIANDER

Source: Coriander consists of the dried ripe fruits of *Coriandrum sativum* L. (Fam. Umbelliferae). It contains not less than 0.3% v/w of volatile oil.

Synonyms and Regional Names: Coriander fruit; Ben. Dhane; Guj. Dhane; Hin. Dhaniya; Kan. Kottambari bija; Mal. Kottam Malli palari; Mar. Kotimbir; San. Dhanyakam; Tam. Kottammali; Tel. Dhaniyalu.

Morphology: Type of fruit – Cremocarp; Shape – subglobular or oval with 5 calyx-teeth and a short stylopod at the apex and some times a short stalk (pedicel) at the base. A cremocarp is made of 2 hemispherical mericarps. Each mericarp has 2 surfaces – a flat surface called the commisural surface and a rounded surface called the dorsal surface. Dorsal surface of each mericarp shows 5 primary and 4 secondary ridges. The primary ridges are wavy, inconspicuous and alternate with prominent, straight secondary ridges. The commisural surface shows the carpophore, a thin elongated structure, attached to the pedicel below and continued upto the upper end of mericarp, and holds both the mericarps together. Size – 2.3 to 4.3 mm(d); Colour – straw yellow or brownish yellow; Odour – aromatic and Taste – spicy and agreeable.

Based on the size of the fruit, two varieties are recognized: *Coriandrum sativum* var. *vulgare macrocarpum* (3 to 5 mm) and *C. sativum* var. *microcarpum* (1.5 to 3 mm).

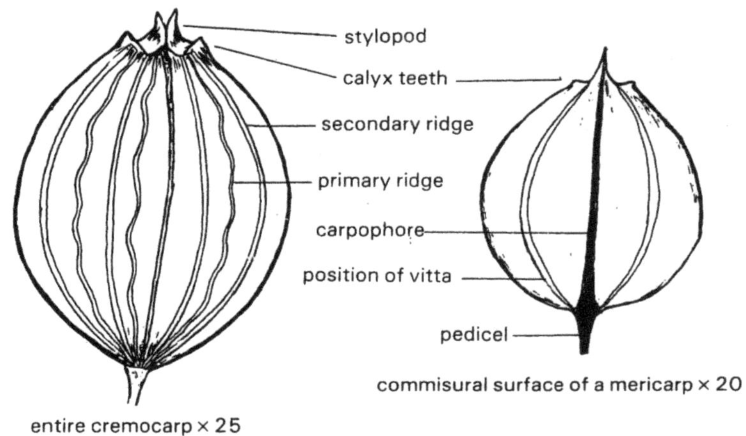

CORIANDER FRUIT

Active Constituents: VOLATILE OIL (0.2 – 1%) – Linalool (60 – 70%) – Terpenes (20%) – Geraniol, Borneol, Citronellol.

Therapeutical and Pharmaceutical Uses:

FATTY OIL (13 – 20%), PROTEIN (17%).

1. Carminative (relieves excessive collection of gas in the stomach).
2. Aromatic and stimulant.

COTTON

Source: Cotton consists of the epidermal trichomes of the seeds of *Gossypium herbaceum* L. and other cultivated species of *Gossypium* (Fam. Malvaceae).

Synonyms and Regional Names: Cotton, Ben. Kapas; Guj. Vona; Hin. Kapas; Kan. Hatti; Mal. Paruti; Mar. Khapus; San. Karpasi; Tam. Paruti; Tel. Paththi.

Chemical Constituents

CARBOHYDRATES – Polysaccharides, Cellulose (90%).
WAX, OIL and FAT in traces.

Therapeutical and Pharmaceutical Uses

1. Main constituent of Surgical Dressings.   2. Filtering Medium.   3. Insulating Material.

Chemical Tests

1. No fumes or odour is liberated when cotton is advanced towards a flame.
2. Blue colour is obtained when cotton is moistened with N/50 iodine and 80% H_2SO_4.

3. Cotton dissolves in cold 80% H_2SO_4.
4. Insoluble in cold sulphuric acid (60%), warm (40%) HCl, 5% KOH, 90% Formic acid, 90% phenol and acetone.
5. Gives no red stain with phloroglucinol and HCl.
6. With ammoniacal copper oxide soln. raw cotton dissolves with ballooning leaving a few fragments of cuticle; absorbent cotton dissolves completely with uniform swelling.

DATURA HERB

Source: Datura Herb consists of the dried leaves and flowering tops of *Datura metel* L. (white variety) *D. metel* var. *fastuosa* (Fam. Solanaceae). It contains not less than 0.20% of total alkaloids of Datura, calculated as hyoscyamine.

Synonyms and Regional Names: *Datura fastuosa* (black variety); Ben. Dhatura; Guj. Dhatoria; Hin. Dhatura; Kan. Kariummathi; Mal. Kariummatham; Mar. Kala dhotari; San. Krishna ummatha; Tam. Karuummattai; Tel. Nallaummatta.

Morphology: *Datura metel* – Sub glabrous spreading herb with cylindrical stem and single triangular ovate leaves, lamina base unequal and leaf margin toothed. Flowers solitary, funnel shaped, large and tubular, 7.5 to 9 cm(l), corolla 15 to 18 cm(l)

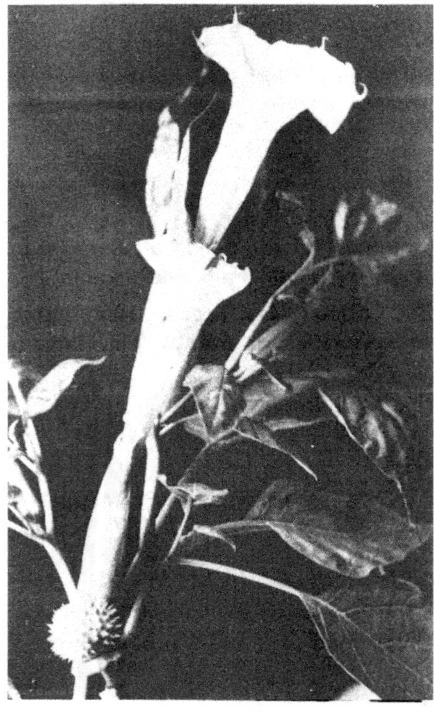

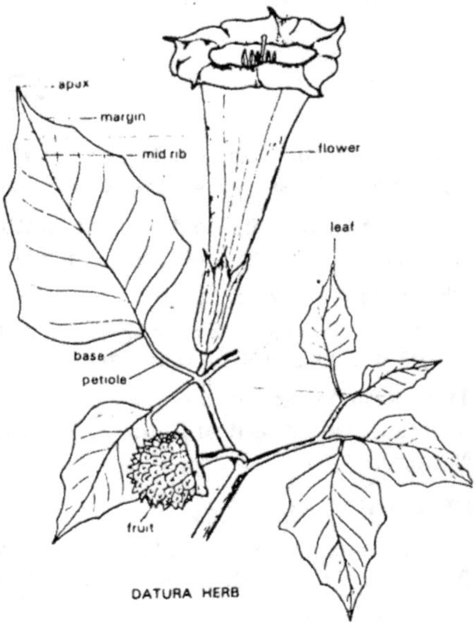

DATURA HERB

10 to 12.5 cm across at the mouth. Fruit a sub-globose capsule covered with short and blunt spines, 2.5 to 3.2 cm(d) nodding or sub-erect. *D. metel* var. *fastuosa.* While many characters of this plant are similar to those of *D. metel* the stem, branches, main veins of leaves and also flowers are violet or purple coloured. Double – flowered and triple flowered forms (outer corolla 5 teeth and inner corolla 6 to 10 teeth) also occur, though not so common.

    D. innoxia also resembles *D. metel* but can be distinguished by the presence of dense pubescence, ovate leaves with cordate base, 10 toothed corolla and long weak spines on the capsular fruit.

Active Constituents: ALKALOIDS (2 – 3%) – Tropane alkaloids – Hyoscyamine
                    FLAVONOIDS   – Scopolamine
                                                    = Hyoscine

Therapeutical and Pharmaceutical Uses

1. Mydriatic (dilation of the pupil).
2. Antispasmodic (counteracts sudden, violent, involuntary muscular contraction).
3. Antimuscarinic effect (acts peripherally to produce parasympathetic inhibition).
4. Antisialagogue (a drug that inhibitis the flow of saliva).
5. Cerebral sedative (reduces excitement).

DIGITALIS

Source: Digitalis is the leaf of *Digitalis purpurea* L. (Fam. Scrophulariaceae) dried at a temperature below 60° immediately after collection.

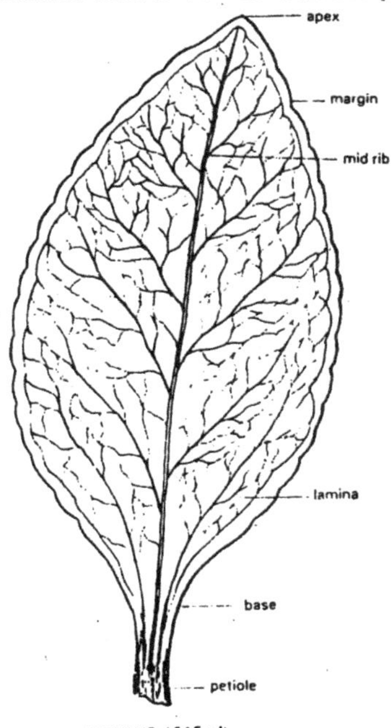

DIGITALIS LEAF × ½

Synonyms and Regional Names
Fox glove,
Digitalis leaf

Morphology
Type – simple;
Size – 10 to 30 cm in length, 4 to 11 cm in width; Shape – ovate lanceolate to broadly ovate;
Petiole – winged;
Margin crenate to· serrate, also dentate. at times;

Apex — obtuse or rounded; Base – tapers into a winged petiole; Venation – pinnate, prominent on the lower surface, close network of veinlets; U. Sur – dark green and minutely hairy; L. Sur – pale green to greyish green and pubescent; Odour – distinct; Taste – very bitter.

Active Constituents: GLYCOSIDES – Cardiac glycosides – Cardenolides.

(Primary glycoside)		(Secondary glyco.)		(Aglycone)
Purpurea glycoside A	(EH)	Digitoxin	(AH)	Digitoxigenin
Purpurea glycoside B	(EH)	Gitoxin	(AH)	Gitoxigenin
Glucogitaloxin	(EH)	Gitaloxin	(AH)	Gitaloxigenin

EH — Enzymic hydrolysis, AH — Acidic hydrolysis.

In the above glycosides the sugars are same. That is the primary glycoside on enzymic hydrolysis yields corresponding secondary glycoside and one molecule of dextrose as the sugar part. Further, when the secondary glycosides undergo acidic hydrolysis, the corresponding aglycones are obtained alongwith 3 molecules of a rare or special sugar called as Digitoxose.

Saponin glycosides – gitonin, digitonin etc.; Flavonoids.

Therapeutical and Pharmaceutical Uses

1. Cardiotonic (having a tonic effect on the heart)
2. Employed in most forms of cardiac failure.
3. Diuretic (stimulates the flow of urine) in cardiac edema.

Chemical Tests: Cardiac glycosides (Cardenolides).

1. Test based on special sugar-Digitoxose, a desoxy sugar. Keller Kiliani Test – Digitoxose (or even cymarose from *Strophanthus kombe)* or the glycoside is dissolved in glacial acetic acid with one or two drops of $FeCl_3$ in it and this is now added to a soln. of conc. H_2SO_4 also containing one or two drops of $FeCl_3$. At the junction of the two layers formed on mixing, reddish brown colour is seen and the upper acetic acid layer turns bluish green.

   The next two tests are based on the presence of 5-membered unsaturated lactone ring – Cardenolides (eg. *D. purpurea, D lanata* and *S. kombe*).
2. Baljet Test: Glycoside/Aglycone + Sodium picrate → yellow to orange colour.
3. Legal Test: Glycoside/Aglycone in pyridine is made alkaline by adding sodium nitroprusside soln. – pink to red colour.

Substitutes and Adulterants: The adulterants of Folia *Digitalis* can be distinguished on the basis of trichomes. While collapsed trichomes are the characteristic features of *D. purpurea* in Mullein leaves which is obtained from *Verbascum thapsus* (Scrophulariaceae), candelabra trichomes which are woolly and branched are noted. in Comfrey leaves (*Symphytum officinale*-Boraginaceae), isolated stiff unicellular trichomes and many of them curved into a hook at the apex are seen. One other adulterant is Primrose leaves obtained from *Primula vulgaris* (Fam. Primulaceae). Here the covering trichomes are uniseriate and four to nine cells long. The short glandular trichomes are with unicellular stalk and a globular unicellular head.

DILL

Source: Dill consists of the dried fruits of *Anethum graveolens* L. (*Anethum sowa* Kurz-Indian Dill) Fam. Umbelliferae. It contains not less than 2.5% of volatile oil.

Synonyms and Regional Names: Ben. Hin. Sowa; Guj. Suva; Kan. Sata; Mal. Katukuppa; Mar. Shepu; San. Sata pushpi; Tam. Sata kupi; Tel. Sompa.

Morphology (INDIAN DILL): Type of Fruit — Cremocarp, market sample comprises of both entire as well separated mericarps. Form — broadly ovate; dorsally compressed and has thin, flat wings. Colour — pale brown to dark brown and some varieties greyish green as well, Surface — yellowish primary ridges, 5 in number, 2 of them are used up for the formation of lateral wings and the other three are feebly developed, Size — 4 mm(l); 2 to 3 mm(w) and 1 mm(t), Odour and taste — characteristic; aromatic and spicy.

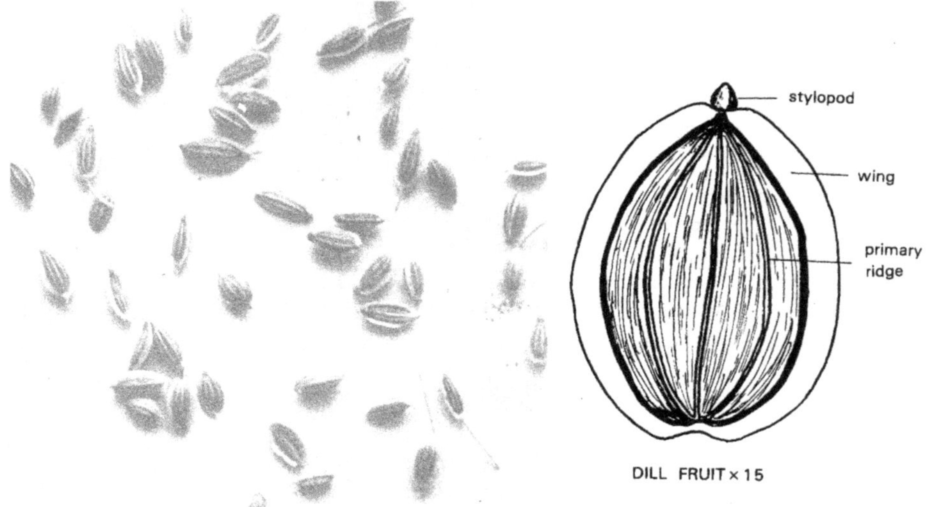

DILL FRUIT × 15

Active Constituents: VOLATILE OIL (3 to 3.5%)

    DILL — Carvone (50 – 60%) – dihydrocarvone in traces, d-limonene, phellandrene

    INDIAN DILL — Dill-apiole (toxic and poisonous) – Carvone (15 to 30%).

— Dihydrocarvone (4 to 12%) and myristicin, thymol and 30 to 40% of hydrocarbons.

Therapeutical Uses: Carminative (eliminates the excessive gas collected in stomach). Used also as a stimulant.

    Indian Dill because of the poisonous substance is not generally used except in veterinary practices.

DIOSCOREA

Source: Dioscorea consists of the tubers of a number of wild and cultivated *Dioscorea* species like *D. deltoidea* Wall, *D. prazeri* Prain & Burkil and *D. floribunda* Mart & Gal. (Fam. Dioscoreaceae).

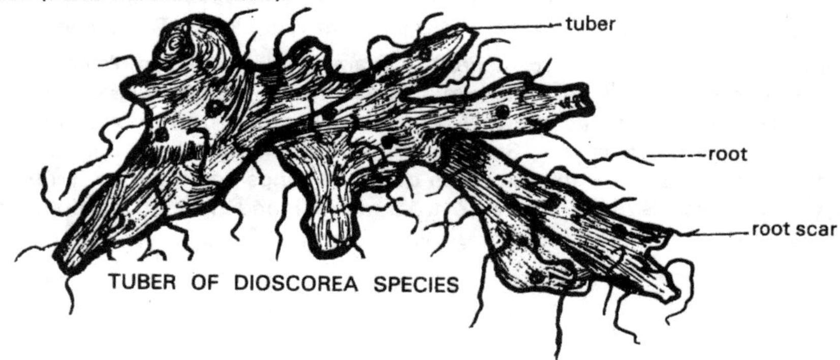

Morphology: Rhizomes of *D. deltoidea* — horizontal tubers, digitate, chestnut brown with recoiling roots; *D. prazeri;* stout horizontal creeping, freely branched,branches about 10 cm(l), 1.5 to 2 cm(w), grey brown-blackish, fresh white or creamy.

Active Constituents

GLYCOSIDES — Saponin glycosides — Steroidal sapogenins.
           — Diosgenin (5% on dry weight basis).
             Glycoside of Prazerigenin
           — a new saponin glycoside with diosgenin and 3 glucose molecules

Therapeutical and Pharmaceutical Use: Steroid precursors.

EPHEDRA

Source: Ephedra consists of the dried young stems of *Ephedra gerardiana* (Wall), Stapf and also of *E. nebrodensis* (Tineo) Stapf, (Fam. Gnetaceae), collected in autumn. Ephedra contains not less than 1.0% of total alkaloids, calculated as ephedrine, $C_{10}H_{15}ON$.

Synonyms and Regional Names: Ma-Huang, Amsania, Butshur, Chewa.

Morphology: Ephedra plant is a small woody dioecious shrub of 1 m height; Size — varies; Colour — older plants straw coloured and younger greyish green; Shape — stems cylindrical and much branched; branches whorled, erect or initially a little spreading and then ascending almost upwards. Nodes and internodes are seen clearly. Surface-main stem is woody and young twigs are slender, however the surfaces of both show striations; Leaves — reduced to minute 2-toothed sheaths. These scaly leaves are brownish to whitish brown, connate opposite and decussate with acute or obtuse apex; Fracture — fibrous in the cortical region whereas pith shows brown powdery mass. Odour — when fresh, the herb is aromatic, no odour

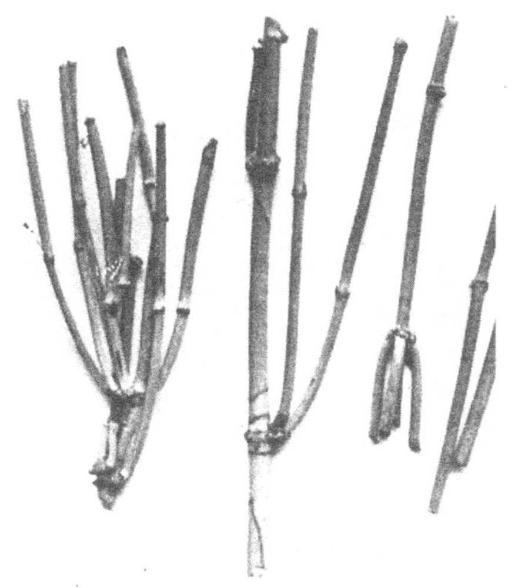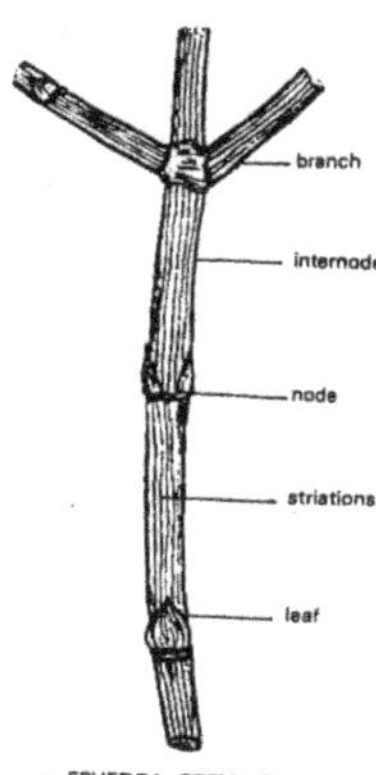

when dry; Taste — bitter and astringent. Based on morphological characters like shape and number or leaves, shape of teeth, number of ridges, length of internodes etc., species differentiation is possible. For instance in *E. nebrodensis,* the leaf apex is acute whereas it is obtuse in the case of *E. gerardiana.*

Active Constituents

ALKALOIDS (0.5 – 3.0%) — Alkaloidal amines – Ephedrine (30 – 90%)
                — Pseudoephedrine – Nor-Pseudoephedrine etc.

Therapeutical and Pharmaceutical Uses

1. Ephedrine is employed in asthmatic conditions and Hay fever (it has an action similar to adrenaline).
2. It produces lasting increase of blood pressure, causes Mydriasis (dilation of the pupil) and diminishes Hyperemia (excess of blood in any part).

Test for Ephedrine: Dissolve 10 mg in 1 ml of water, add 0.2 ml of dil. HCl and 0.1 ml of Copper sulphate soln. followed by 1 ml of sodium hydroxide soln. The resulting solution turns violet. Add 1 ml of solvent ether and shake; the ethereal layer will turn purple and the aqueous layer blue.

ERGOT

Source: Ergot is the dried sclerotium of *Claviceps purpurea* (Fries). Tulasne (Fam. Hypocreaceae) developed on Rye plants, *Secale cereale* L (Fam. Graminae). It contains not less than 0.19% of the total alkaloids of Ergot, calculated as ergotoxine, of which not less than 15.0% consists of water soluble alkaloids of Ergot, calculated as ergometrine.

Synonym and Regional Name: Ergot of Rye
                         Secale cornutum

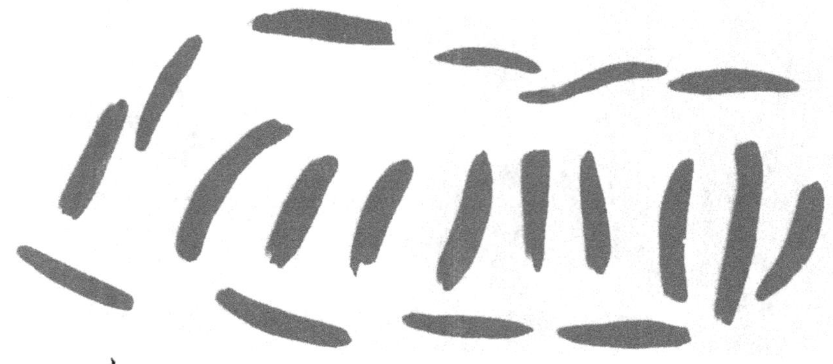

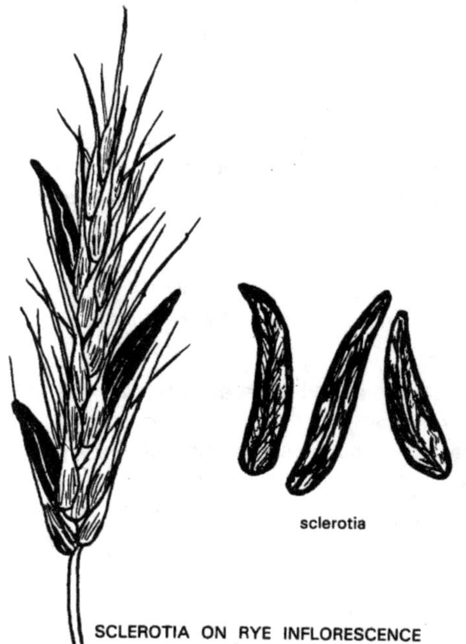

sclerotia

SCLEROTIA ON RYE INFLORESCENCE

Morphology

Sclerotium: Shape — fusiform, slightly curved, tapering towards both ends, occasionally straight, 3 or 4 sided; Colour — dark violet to black; Size — 1.5 to 4 cm(l) and 2 to 7 mm(b); Surface — longitudinal furrows and transverse cracks conspicuous on the concave side; Fracture — short, fractured surface shows a thin dark purple outer layer of tissues and a whitish or pinkish white, central zone with darker lines radiating from the centre; Odour — faint and characteristic; Taste — characteristic and unpleasant.

Active Constituents: ALKALOIDS — Indole type (0.1 to 0.8%).

1. Water soluble
   Ergometrine grp.
   Ergometrine
   Ergometrinine

2. Water Insoluble (ether soluble)

a) Ergotamine grp.
   Ergotamine
   Ergotaminine
   Ergosine
   Ergosinine

b) Ergotoxine grp.
   Ergocristine
   Ergocristinine
   Ergocryptine
   Ergocryptinine
   Ergocornine
   Ergocorninine

Further, all alkaloids are derivatives of either lysergic acid or isolysergic acid. In the *Ergometrine* alkaloids, lysergic acid or its isomer is linked to an *Amino alcohol.* The water insoluble alkaloids are polypeptides in which lysergic acid or its isomer is linked to *Amino acids.* If the amino acids involved in Ergotamine group are for instance XYZ, the amino acids in Ergotoxine group are XMZ. Only the lysergic acid derivatives (d – series) whose words end in 'ine' are active. The alkaloid derivatives (d-series) whose words end in 'nine' are inactive. Though the proportion of different groups is different in different races of ergot, the polypeptides are more than the other group.

Prof. Wagner of West Germany however presents the chemical constituents in a different way. According to him around 30 alkaloids are known to occur and these are classified chiefly into two groups – (a) *Lysergic acid* (therp. important) alkaloids and (b) *Clavine alkaloids* (therp. not important). The basic ring for both types is 'ergoline'. The lysergic acid alkaloids are further divided into two groups – (a) Acid amide alkaloids – Ergometrine.. water soluble (b) Peptide alkaloids – Ergotamine and Ergotoxine – water insoluble.

Besides the drug also contains 30% fat which in turn contains about 35% Ricinoleic acid ester. The cell walls are chitinous in nature.

Therapeutical Uses
1. Oxytocic (hastens the child delivery) – Ergometrine grp.
2. Antiepinephrine activity (an agent that neutralizes the action of adrenaline only) – Ergotamine grp.
3. In the treatment of persistent migraine (a type of headache).
4. Sympathicolytic (a drug that neutralizes the action of sympathetic nervous system).

Storage: Ergot is eaten by insects, moulds and bacteria. After collection it should be thoroughly dried, kept entire and stored in a cool place. If powdered and not immediately defatted the activity decreases, but if defatted and carefully stored in an airtight container, it will remain active for a long period. Bad sample of ergot deteriorates completely.

Chemical Test: *Ergot alkaloids* – Apply a spot of an extract of ergot dissolved in chloroform to a piece of filter paper and allow to dry. Spray with 1% soln. of p – dimethylamino-benzaldehyde in a mixutre of equal parts of ethanol and HCl and warm the paper in hot air. Ergot alkaloids and LSD give a purple colour.

EUCALYPTUS

Source: Eucalyptus is the scythe shaped leaf of *Eucalyptus globulus* Labill & *E. citriodora* Hook. (Fam. Myrtaceae). Oil of Eucalyptus is the volatile oil obtained by steam distillation from the fresh leaves of *E. globulus,* and rectified.

Synonyms and Regional Names: Hin. Neeli-gond ka tel; Mal. Karpuramaram; Tam. Karpuramarat thailam; Tel. Talanoppi.

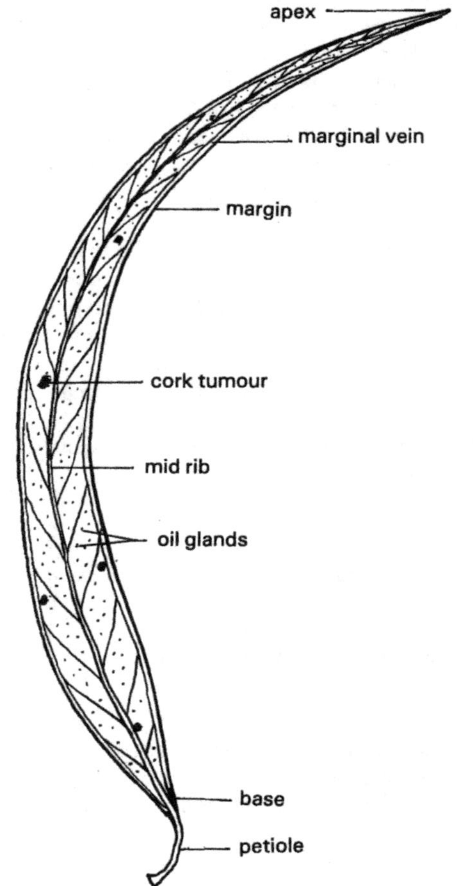

Morphology: Form – lanceolate, scythe shaped sessile or petiolate; Colour – greyish green; Surface – glabrous with characteristic marginal vein, thin and wax coated; Nature of Oil: Colour – colourless or pale yellow liquid, Odour – aromatic camphoraceous; Taste – pungent, camphoraceous and cool feeling.

Active Constituents: VOLATILE OIL (3 to 6%) – Eucalyptol/ Cineole – an oxide, piperitone, phellandrene, geraniol – geranyl aceate – citronellal.

Gallo tannins, methyl ester of p-coumaric acid, a dihydro flavonol aromadendrin – 7-methyl ether and cinnamic acid in combined form. CITRIODOROL (from *E. citriodora*).

Therapeutical and Pharmaceutical Uses
1. Antiseptic, anti-bacterial and anti-tuberculosis (citriodorol).
2. Diaphoretic.
3. Expectorant.

FENNEL

Source: Fennel consists of the dried ripe fruits of *Foeniculum vulgare* Mill. (Fam. Umbelliferae), from cultivated plants. It contains not less than 1.4% v/w of volatile oil

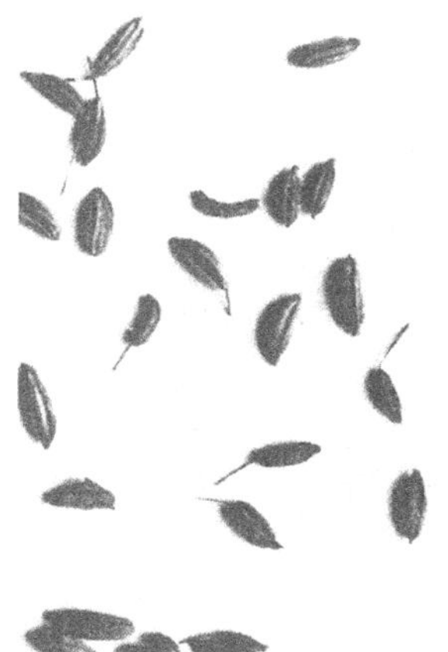

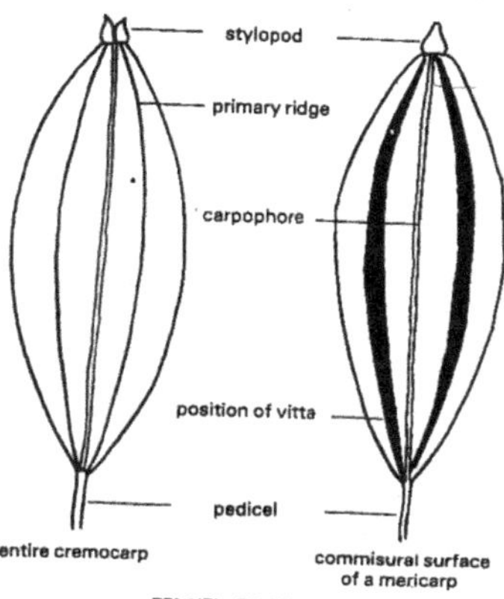

Morphology: Type – Cremocarp with two one-seeded mericarps; Shape – straight or slightly curved, oblong, laterally compressed, tapering towards the base and apex. At the apex a short curved bifid structure called as stylopod is present. A thin pedicel is seen at the base; Size — 5 to 10 mm(l), 2 to 4 mm(b); Surface – each mericarp has two surfaces-the dorsal and the commisural surface. Dorsal surface is glabrous with 5 straight, prominent primary ridges and stylopod at the apex. Commisural surface is flat and shows the carpophore which holds the two mericarps together; Colour – greenish or yellowish brown; Odour and Taste – strongly aromatic.

Microscopy (Transverse Section)

Fennel exhibits features of a typical unbelliferous fruit – CREMOCARP. When a *schizocarp* (a fruit which splits apart into parts but without further dehiscion) is derived from a bicarpellary pistil, it is called a *cremocarp.* In otherwords, a cremocarp consists of two portions each of which is called a *mericarp* connected by a central stalk called carpophore. A single seed is seen in each mericarp.

T.S. of mericarp shows two prominent surfaces – the commisural and the dorsal. The commisural surface is flat with two pronounced ridges and carpophore in the middle. The dorsal surface is also ridged (3 ridges). Thus, in all, the mericarp shows 5 primary ridges.

Mericarp can broadly be divided into Pericarp, Testa and the bulky Endosperm. **PERICARP:** The *Epicarp* or the exocarp of the pericarp surrounding the entire mericarp consists of a layer of polygonal, tangentially elongated cells with smooth cuticle.

MESOCARP: The bulk of mesocarp is made of parenchyma, Bicollateral vascular bundles appear in the mesocarp below the primary ridges. *Reticulate and lignified parenchyma,* a characteristic feature of Fennel appears in the mesocarp surrounding the vascular bundles. Besides, yellowish brown and elliptical vittae (schizogenous oil ducts), 4 on the dorsal surface between the ridges and two on the commisural surface are also important features of mesocarp.

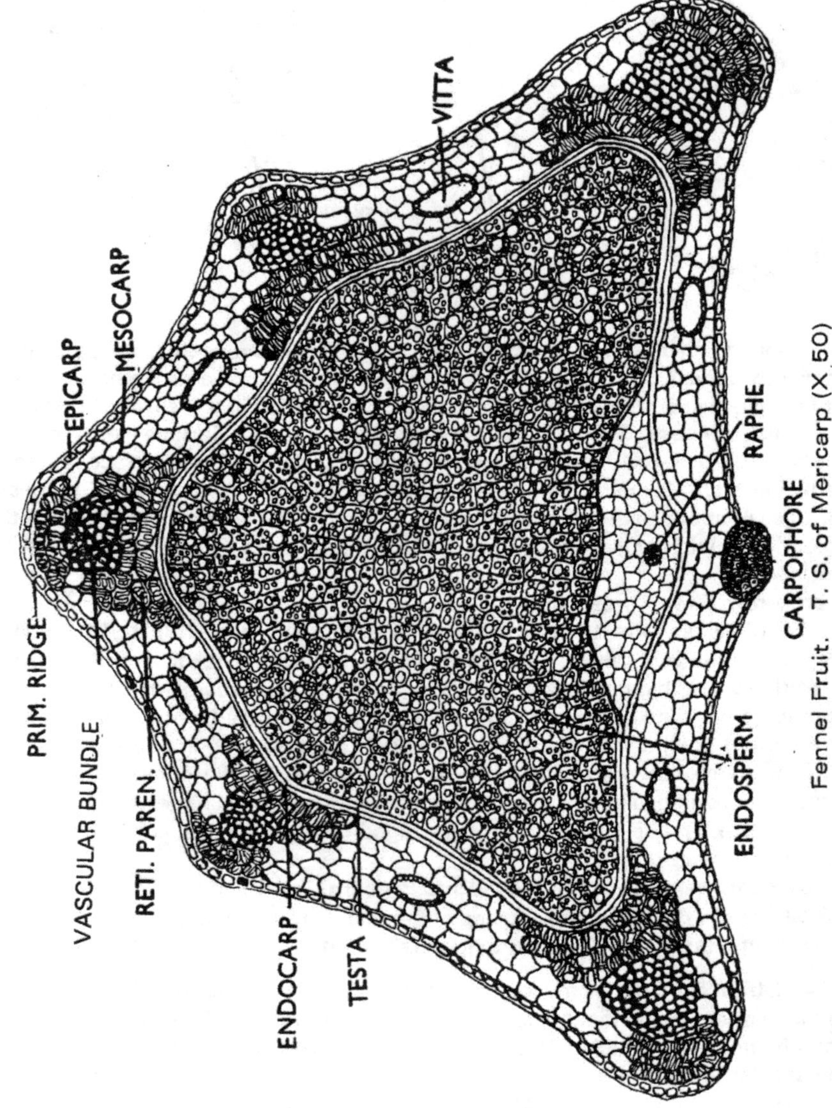

Fennel Fruit. T. S. of Mericarp (X. 50)

Endocarp: Another typical umbelliferous feature is the presence of *parquetry arrangement* (groups of parallel cells arranged in different directions) of cells of endocarp which however is seen as a single layer between mesocarp and testa.

TESTA single layered and yellowish in colour.

ENDOSPERM thick walled, polygonal colourless parenchyma containing oil globules and aleurone grains. A crescent shaped embryo is seen in the sections passing through the apical region of mesocarp Raphe, a ridge of vascular strand, appears in the middle of commisural surface just in front of carpophore, as the ovule is anatropous (inverted) here.

Active Constituents: VOLATILE OIL (4 – 6%) – Anethole (50 – 60%), a phenolic ether – d-Fenchone (20%), a ketone – Methyl chavicol, terpineol etc.
FATTY OIL (12 – 18%) and PROTEIN (14 – 22%) are also present, though not active.

Therapeutical and Pharmaceutical Uses: 1. Spasmolytic, 2. Carminative, 3. Stomachic (gastric stimulant), 4. Appetizer, 5. Galactagogue (increases the flow of milk) 6. Comforts the belly ache in infants 7. Eye wash (Aqua Foeniculi).

Substitutes and Adulterants: Like other volatile oil drugs, here too the exhausted Fennel is an adulterant. The oil may be removed partly or completely either by steam distillation as usual or by solvent extraction using a solvent like alcohol. Fennel subjected to steam distillation will be darker in colour and shrunken in appearance. Alcohol exhausted Fennel will have a fusel – oil odour (nauseous oil in spirits distilled from potatoes, grain etc.). Further the exhausted fennel will sink in water.

GELATIN

Source: Gelatin is a product obtained by the partial hydrolysis of collagen, derived from the skin, white connective tissues and bones of animals.

Nature: Occurs in thin sheets, strips or as granular powder. High grade gelatin is light yellow, semi-crystalline substance without any odour or taste. Solubility: in cold water it swells up and slowly dissolves on warming to form viscous soln.

Chemical Constituents: Protein – Glutin – Amino acids.

Therapeutical and Pharmaceutical Uses: 1. In capsule preparations 2. In making suppositories 3. As culture medium in Bacteriology 4. Source of Protein in nutritional experiments. 5. As a substitute for blood plasma 6. Zinc oxide is added to form zinc gelatin which is used in topical protectant.

Chemical Tests

1. Ammonia is evolved when heated with soda-lime. powder.
   Preparation of the test soln.
   Dissolve 0.5 g of Gelatin in 100 ml water by heating and use this soln. for the following tests –
2. On addition of Millon's reagent to a few ml of the test soln., a white ppt. is produced which turns red on heating.
3. To 1 ml of test soln. add 1 ml of 10% mercuric sulphate in 10% sulphuric acid. Boil gently for 30 sec. Add 2 drops of 1% sodium nitrite soln. Red ppt. or colour is obtained.
4. Biuret Test: To 3 ml of test soln. NaoH (1 ml of 5%) is added to make it strongly alkaline – A violet or pink colour is developed on addition of 2 drops of 1% $CuSO_4$.
5. To a few ml of test soln. few drops of 10% Tannic acid is added whereby white to whitish buff coloured ppt. is formed which does not dissolve on heating.
6. Yellow ppt. is formed on adding picric acid to test soln.
   These above tests distinguish Gelatin from Agar. In Agar these tests are negative.

GENTIAN

Source: Gentian is the dried rhizome and root of *Gentiana lutea* L. (Fam. Gentianaceae).

Synonyms and Regional Names: Gentian root, Bitter root; Ben. Karu, Kutki; Guj. Pakhanbed; Hin. Karu, Kutki.

Morphology: Shape – cylindrical, sometimes longitudinally split; Colour – yellowish brown; Size – varies upto 60 cm (l) and 4 cm (t); Surface – crowded leaf scars

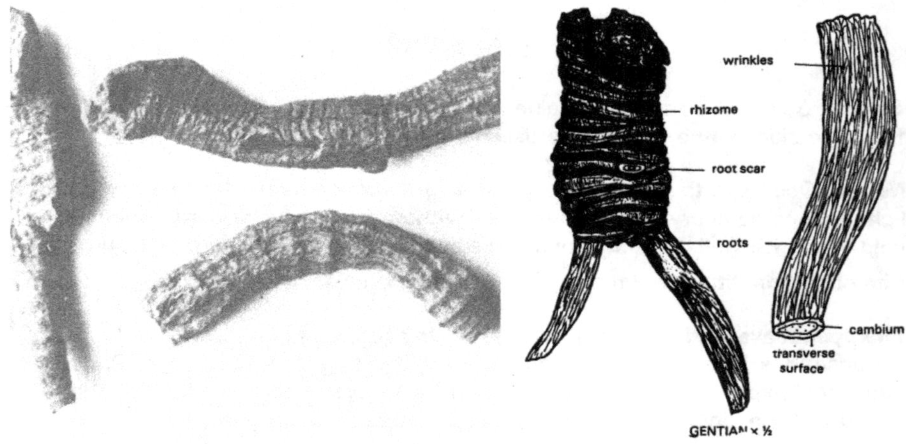

encircle rhizome, whereas longitudinal wrinkles may be seen on the root, Fracture of the dried drug-short; Odour – characteristic and Taste – sweet to start with but later persistently bitter.

Active Constituents: BITTER PRINCIPLES – Gentiopikrin, Amarogentin
ALKALOID (0.6 – 0.8%) – Gentianine
XANTHONE DERIVATIVES – Gentisin, Gentioside
SUGARS – Gentiobiose, Gentianose.

Therapeutical and Pharmaceutical Uses:.1. Bitter tonic.   2. In cases of Anorexie (loss of appetite).   3. Dyspepsia (indigestion). The drug has to be taken 60 to 30 min. before food as the activity of the durg starts only after a latent period.

GINGER

Source: Ginger is the rhizome of *Zingiber officinale Roscoe;* (Fam. Zingiberaceae), scraped to remove the dark outer skin and dried in the sun.

Synonyms and Regional Names: Ben. Ada; Guj. Ale; Hin. Adrak; Kan. Shunti; Mal. Inchi; Mar. Ale; San. Adrakam; Tam. Inji, Sukku; Tel. Sonti, Allamu.

Morphology: Form – irregularly branched (sympodial), laterally compressed, branches known as fingers arise obliquely from the rhizome, 1 to 3 cm(l) and terminate in

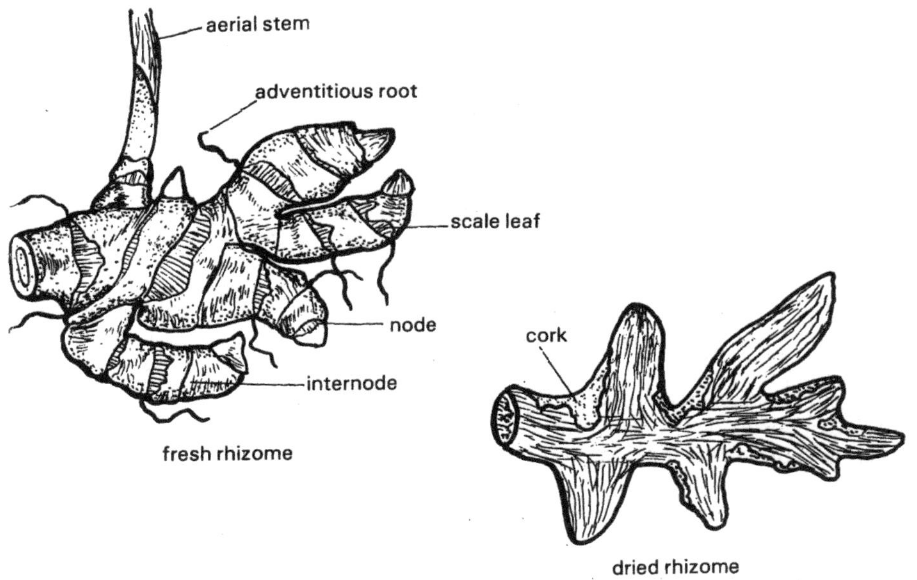

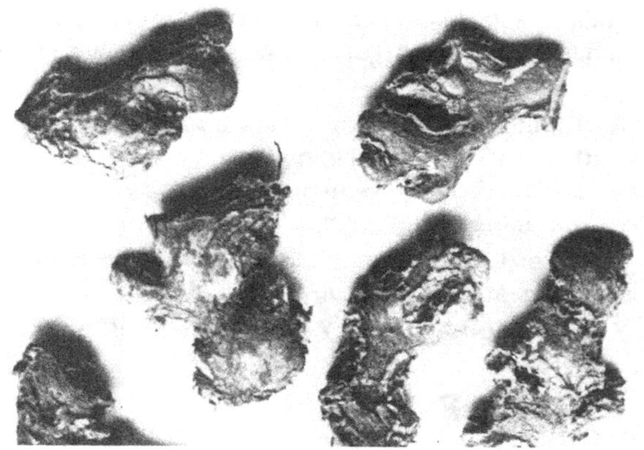

depressed scars or in undeveloped buds. The nodes, internodes and. scales, conspicuous features of fresh samples are not clearly seen in the dried ones; Colour – buff; Size – 7 to 15 cm(l), 3 to 6 cm(w) and 1 to 1.5 cm(t):

Surface – longitudinal striations are seen; Fracture – short, mealy and fibrous Fractured surface shows projecting fibres, Odour – agreeable and aromatic and Taste – pungent.

Microscopy (Transverse Section)

A cross-section of an unpeeled mature rhizome broadly consists of the following tissues from the periphery to the centre.

CORK

Outer cork few layered, dark brown in colour, made of irregular parenchymatous cells.

Inner cork few layered, colourless parenchymatous cells radially arranged in regular rows.

CORTEX thin parenchymatous cells with intercellular spaces containing abundant starch. The starch grains are unique in the sense that they are sack shaped with terminal beak like projection in which the eccentric hilum is situated. Distinct striations are very prominent on the grain. Interspersed with cortical parenchyma are found numerous oleo-resin cells and as well vascular bundles. The oleo-resin cells have suberized walls and contain yellowish matter.

EDODERMIS single layered with radial walls thickened and with no starch grains

GROUND TISSUE large, parenchymatous (similar to that of cortex) with abundant starch, oleo-resin cells and vascular bundles. The latter in general are collateral, conjoint and closed. A group of sclerenchymatous fibres partially covers the vascular bundles of cortex and also of central ground tissue and these bundles are therefore called as Fibrovascular bundles. Just below the endodermal layer, that is to the periphery of the ground tissue, a ring of narrow zone of vascular bundles appear, which however are not covered by sclerenchymatous fibres.

While the *Phloem* presents the usual well-developed sieve elements, *xylem elements* are somewhat characteristic. Xylem consists of mainly vessels, some tracheids which have annular, spiral or reticulate thickenings but without any reaction for lignin. The fibres are also unusually unlignified, pitted and septate.

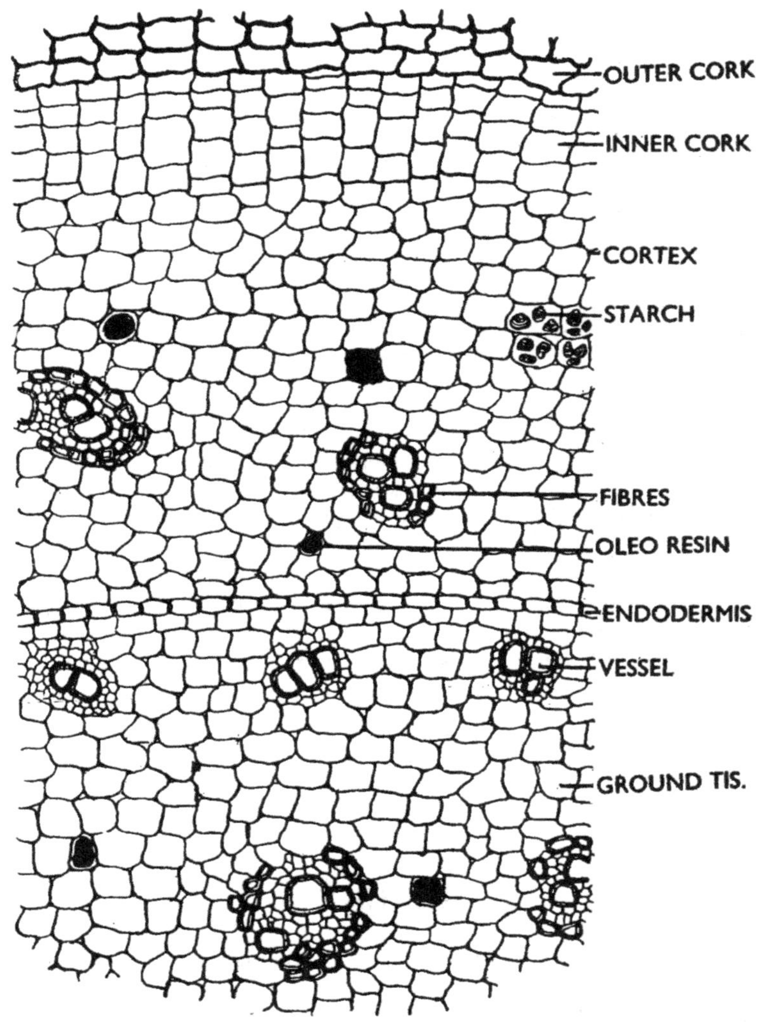

Ginger Rhizome-an enlarged portion of T. S. (X 100)

Active Constituents: VOLATILE OIL (0.6 to 3%) – Sesquiterpene – Zingiberene – Sesquiterpene Alcohol – Zingiberol – Borneol – Linalool, Geraniol etc – Aldehyde-Citral.

PUNGENT PRINCIPLES (5 to 8%) – Gingerol – Shogaol – Zingerone.
Resinous Matter – starch – mucilage.

Therapeutical and Pharmaceutical Uses: 1. Carminative . 2. Stimulant
3. Flavouring agent.

Substitutes and Adulterants: Many books in the field report two common
adulterants.

1. Japanese Ginger is derived from *Zingiber mioga.* Volatile oil has different physical
   properties and the starch grains are compound in nature. In India however, there
   is no fear of this ginger getting mixed up or being used as an adulterant.
2. Exhausted ginger. Powdered Ginger will be subjected to steam distillation or
   extraction. This exhausted ginger or spent ginger will show all the microscopic
   details like starch, vessels, fibres etc. and therefore based on these it is difficult
   to detect. But then as a result of distillation, certain extractives and ash values
   change and only when all factors are taken into consideration, the purity of the
   sample can be made out. The official standards prescribed are: 1. Ash. Total
   ash value should not be more than 6%. Coated ginger, or ginger which
   is not well washed will show more ash value. 2. Water soluble ash should
   not be less than 1.7%. In water extracted drug, the value is as low as
   0.5%. 3. Water soluble extractive is not less than 10%. Water exhausted
   ginger has 6% extractive. Alcohol extracted sample will escape this
   test. 4. 90% alcohol soluble extractive is not less than 4.5%. Ginger
   exhausted with alcohol has 1.5% likewise water exhausted sample escapes
   this test. Sometimes Capsicum or the seeds of Paradise grains which are
   obtained from *Aframomum melegueta* (Zingiberaceae) are added to intensify
   the pungency. The presence of capsicum or paradise grains can be detected
   by boiling with alkali when the pungency of ginger is lost but not those of
   capsicum and paradise grains.

GOKHRU

Source: Gokhru consists of the fruits of *Tribulus terrestris* Linn. (Fam. Zygophyceae).

Synonyms and Regional Names: Calthrop, Caltrap; Ben. Gokhru, Gokshura; Guj.
Betagokhru, Gokharu; Hin. Chhota-Gokhru; Kan. Negalu; Mal. Neringil; Mar.
Gokharu; San. Gokhura, Gokshura; Tam. Nerunji; Tel. Palleru.

Morphology: Form – globose, consisting of usually 5 hairy, often muriculate, woody
cocci, each with 2 very sharp rigid spines and 2 shorter ones. Seeds several in each
coccus, with transverse partitions between them.

Active Constituents: GLYCOSIDES – Saponin glycosides – steroid saponins and
steroid sapogenins – Furostanol bis glycoside protodiosin which on acid hydrolysis

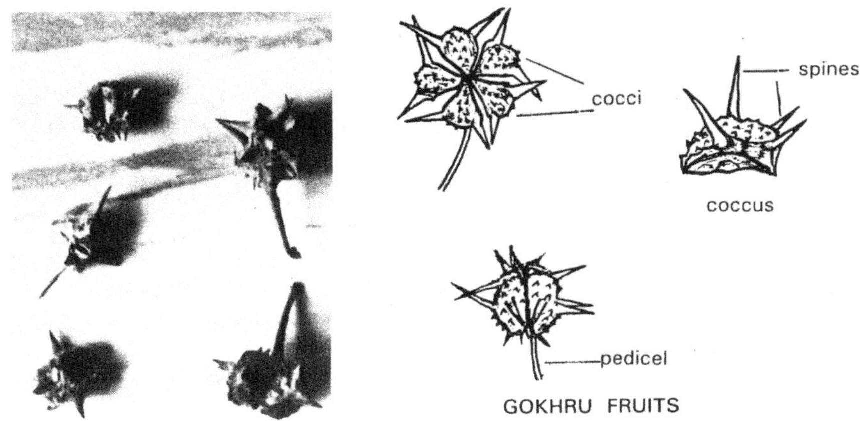

yields the Spirostanol diosgenin, a trace of tigogenin, glucose and rhamnose; — Hecogenin — Neotigogenin.

Therapeutical and Pharmaceutical Uses
1. Diuretic.
2. Cooling tonic and aphrodisiac.
3. In painful micturition (urination), Calculous affections, urinary discharges and impotence.
4. Gokhru is used in 65 drug preparations (Kapoor & Mitra).

GUAR GUM

Source: Guar Gum is obtained from the refined endosperm of the seed of *Cyamopsis tetragonolobus* L. Taub. (Fam. Leguminosae).

Synonym: Guar Cellupectinoid.

Active Constituents: CARBOHYDRATE
Gums — Guaran, the water soluble portion of the gum and yields on hydrolysis galactose 35% and mannose 60 to 65%.

Therapeutical and Pharmaceutical Uses:
1. As a protective colloid.
2. As binding and disintegrating agent in tablet formulations.
3. In bulk laxatives.
4. As appetite depressent.
5. In peptic ulcer therapy.

HONEY

Source: Honey is a sugary secretion deposited in the honey comb by the bee *Apis dorsata* and possibly other species of *Apis*, eg. *Apis indica, A. florea* etc. (Fam. Apidae).

Synonyms and Regional Names: Honey, Ben. Modh; Guj. (Mar.) Madh; Hin. (San.) Madhu; Kan. Jenu tuppa; Mal. (Tam.) Ten; Tel. Tene.

Nature: Viscous, translucent liquid, Colour – yellowish to dark brown; Odour – agreeable; Taste – sweet; Solubility – soluble in water and alcohol.

Chemical Constituents: CARBOHYDRATES – Invert sugars 70 – 80% (equimolar mixture of dextrose and fructose), sucrose (0.1 – 10%).

Enzymes, vitamins, micro elements and mineral substances and organic acids.

Therapeutical and Pharmaceutical Uses

1. As a pharmaceutical aid.
2. Nutrient and demulcent (soothing).
3. Laxative.
4. As a pill excipient (in the preparation of pills).

Chemical Tests

1. Test for reducing sugars – 0.5 g of honey is dissolved in 10 ml of water and boiled after adding Fehling's soln. A heavy red ppt. of copper oxide is seen indicating the presence of reducing sugars.
2. **Selivanoff's Test**: To the test soln. a crystal of resorcinol is added and also equal volume of con. HCl. On warming over a water bath, ketoses like honey, fructose etc., give rose colour.
3. Detection – 1 ml of honey is mixed with 4 ml of alcohol whereby more than a slight turbidity indicates the presence of dextrin from added glucose.
4. Fiehe's test to detect adulteration – Artificial invert sugar sucrose and commercial liquid glucose are used as adulterants of honey. Release of furfural, which is not present in the natural honey, on acidic hydrolysis is detected in this test:

    10 ml of honey is shaken thoroughly with 5 ml of ether till they are miscible and later separate on standing. The upper ethereal layer is evaporated to dryness in a porcelain dish. In natural honey, a transient red colouration is obtained on addition of 1 drop 1% resorcinol HCl while in artificial invert sugar, red colouration persists for sometime.

HYOSCYAMUS

Source: Hyoscyamus consists of the dried leaves, or leaves and flowering tops, of *Hyoscyamus niger* L. (Fam. Solanaceae). It contains not less than 0.05% of the alkaloids of Hyoscyamus, calculated as hyoscyamine.

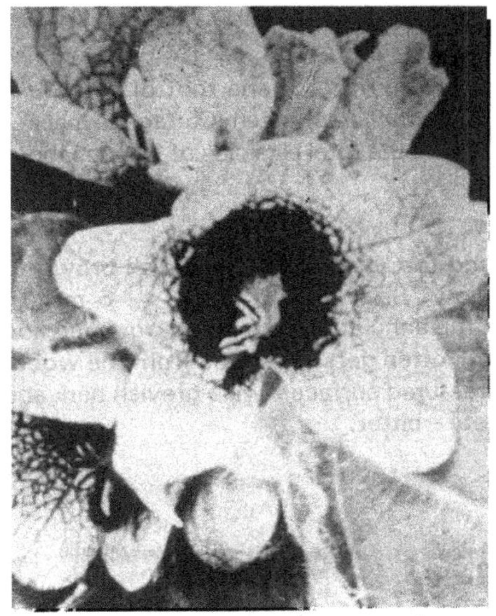 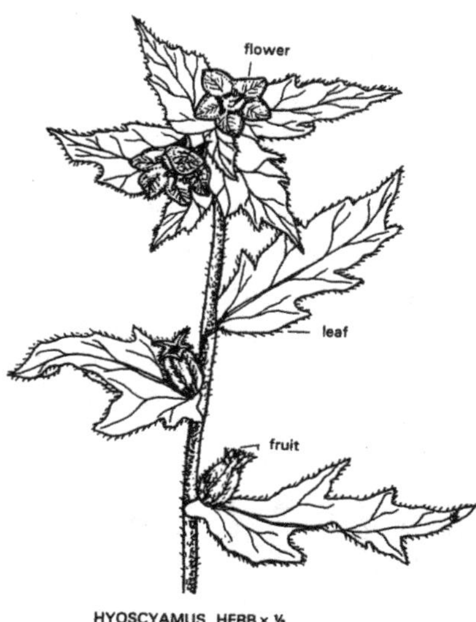

Synonyms and Regional Names: Henbane, Stinking night shade; Ben. Guj. Hin. Khorasani ajowan; San. Parasikaya, Kurasani, Yamani; Tam. Tel. Kurasaniyomam.

Morphology of the Herb: Leaves: Type – simple; Shape – ovate, oblong to triangular ovate, Size of lamina – 30 cm(l) margin – irregularly dentate, apex – acute; Venation – pinnate; Surface – glandular and hairy; Colour – light greyish green, Texture – soft and sticky, Odour – strong and characteristic; Taste – bitter and acrid. Flowers: – Colour – yellow with purple veins; Size – 1.5 cm(l), 2.5 cm(d), calyx – 5 lobed peristent, corolla – funnel shaped and 5 lobed, ovary – superior. Fruit: size – 1 cm(l); Shape – ovoid – oblong. Type – pyxis, encircled by the calyx which protrudes above the fruit; Seeds: numerous, reniform in shape and 1 mm(l), seed coat – brown and reticulate.

Active Constituents
ALKALOIDS – Tropane alkaloids (0.04 – 0.72%)

– Hyoscyamine (60%) – Scopolamine = Hyoscine (40%), Atropine, Apoatropine, Cuskhygrine

FLAVONOIDS

Therapeutical and Pharmaceutical Uses

1. Mydriatic (dilation of the pupil).
2. Antispasmodic (arrests the involuntary muscular contraction).
3. Antimuscarinic effect (acts peripherally to produce parasympathetic inhibition).
4. Antisialagogue (a drug that arrests the flow of excess of saliva).
5. Cerebral sedative (reduces excitement).

IPECAC

Source: Ipecac consists of the dried root, or the rhizome and root of *Cephaelis ipecacuanha* (Brot) A. Rich. (Rio Ipecac) or *C. acuminata* Karsten (Cartagena Ipecac) (Fam. Rubiaceae). It contains not less than 2% of the total alkaloids of Ipecac, about 50% of which should be emetine.

Synonym: Ipecacuanha.

Morphology: Shape – roughly cylindrical and tortuous; Colour – reddish brown to dark brown, inner wood is however yellow; Size – 5 – 15 cm(l), 4 – 6 mm(t); Surface – closely annulated externally and the annulations are broad, rounded and completely encircle the root. Annulated bark often gets separated from the wood; Fracture – short (bark), splintery (wood); Fractured surface – wide greyish bark and small dense wood, Odour – slight and Taste – bitter.

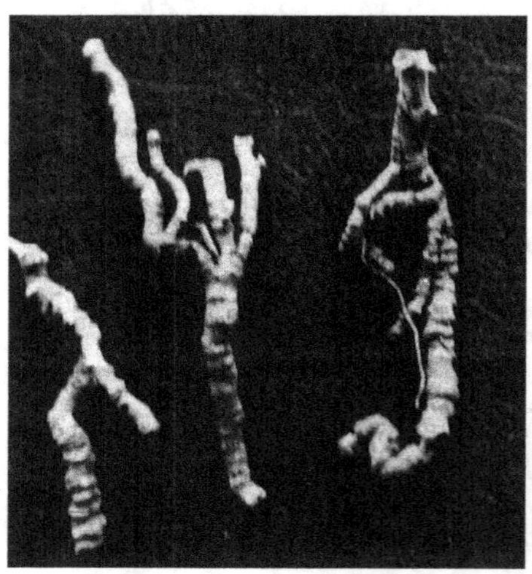

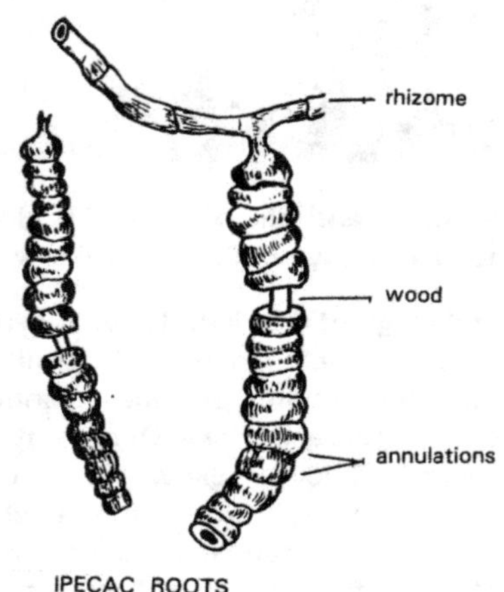

IPECAC ROOTS

Active Constituents: ALKALOIDS – Isoquinoline alkaloids (2 to 6%)
        – Emetine (1.4 – 1.7%) – Cephaeline (0.5 – 1.2%)
        – Psychotrine (0.05%)
        – Psychotrine methylether and – Emetamine.

Test for Emetine: To 0.5 g of the powdered Ipecac add 20 ml HCl and 5 ml water. Filter and to the filtrate add 0.01 g of potassium chlorate; formation of yellow colour is due to emetine.

Therapeutical and Pharmaceutical Uses

1. In cases of amoebic dysentery.
2. Expectorant in dry bronchitis.
3. Emetic (causes vomiting).

Substitutes and Adulterants: Frequent suggestions have appeared in literature as to the use of the following plants as substitutes of Ipecac. None of these however contain emetine or the other alkaloids of Ipecac but then they do contain certain irritant principles which are responsible for the emetic property.

1. *Naregamia alata* (Goanese Ipecac) Meilaceae and contains naregamine.
2. *Cryptocoryne spiralis* (Araceae).
3. *Tylophora asthmatica* (Asclepiadaceae) contains tylophorine and tylophorinine.
4. Bastard Ipecac or Wild Ipecac — *Asclepias curassavica,* (Asclepiadaceae) and contains a glycoside asclepin.

The common adulterants are the Ipecac stems when in excess and *Cephalis undulata.* Ipecac stems also contain the same alkaloids as roots but in lesser concentrations. Morphologically stems are slender, longitudinally striated and show no annulations. In t.s. the stem shows thin bark, á ring of wood and a distinct pith. 2. *C.undulata* has no emetine, roots appear twisted with violet coloured starchy bark.

IPOMOEA

Source: Ipomoea is the dried root of *Ipomoea orizabensis* Ledennois (Fam. Convolvulaceae).

Synonyms: *Convolvulus scammonia,* Orizaba Jalap, Mexican Scammony.

Morphology: Shape — irregular brown pieces or oblique slices; Colour — dark greyish brown (external) and yellowish brown (internal); Size — varies, but usually 3 – 6 cm(w) and upto 4 cm(t); Fracture — very fibrous; Odour — slight and Taste — faintly acrid.

Active Constituents

RESINS (15%) — glycosidal resins (6 – 18%) — Jalapin — Ipuranol, Ipurganol.

— Orizabin, the ether soluble component yields after alkaline hydrolysis glycoside acids — orizabin acid A & B. Acidic hydrolysis of both acids yield Jalapinol acid, glucose, rhamnose, chinovose and fucose. The difference between the two however is only quantitative proportion of sugars (H. Wagner-Drogen und ihre Inhaltstoffe 1979).

VOLATILE OIL, SCOPOLETIN etc.

Therapeutical and Pharmaceutical Use: A strong cathartic.

ISAPGOL

Source: Isapgol consists of the dried seeds of *Plantago ovata* Forsk (Fam. Plantaginaceae).

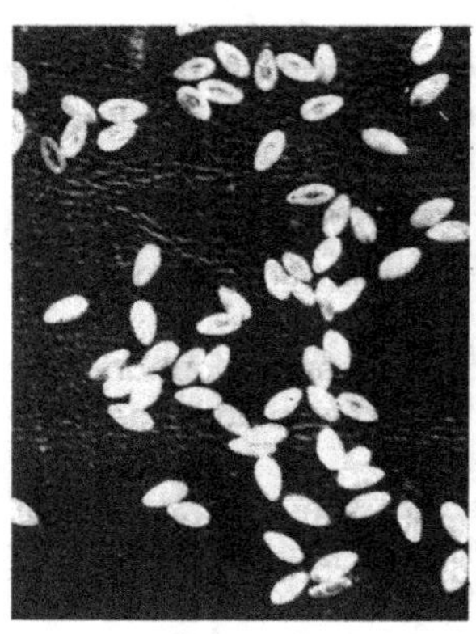
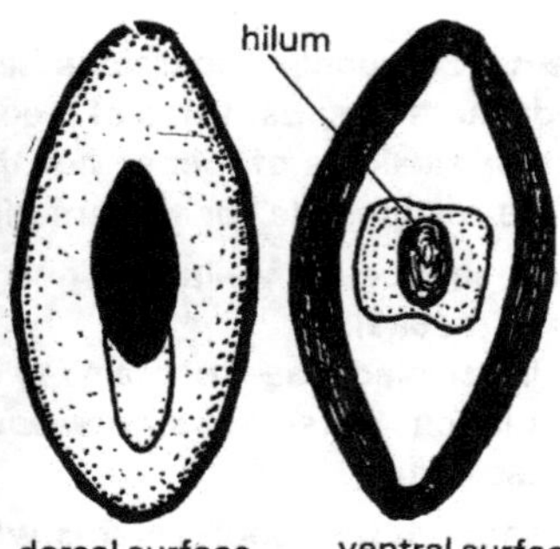

ISAPGOL SEEDS × 20

Morphology: Size — 1 to 3.5 mm(l) and 1 to 1.75 mm(w); Shape — ovate and boat shaped with a dorsal or convex surface and a ventral or concave surface. D. sur. — dull, opaque, pinkish grey, there is a small elongated reddish brown spot in the centre; V. sur — A deep furrow may be seen, Hilum which is covered by thin membrane appears as a red spot in the centre; Odour — none and Taste — mucilaginous

Active Constituents

CARBOHYDRATES — Mucilage (pentosan + Aldobionic acid)

Pentosan — hyd → xylose + arabinose

Aldobionic acid — hyd → galacturonic acid + rhamnose

FIXED OIL and PROTEINS

Therapeutical and Pharmaceutical Uses

1. Demulcent (soothing property).
2. In chronic constipation.
3. In chronic dysentery of amoebic and bacillary origin.
4. In chronic diarrhoeas.

The quality of the drug is based on the mucilage content which is expressed as 'swelling factor'. The principle involved here is that the mucilage in the seed absorbs water and swells. The reading is taken after a stipulated time. The swelling factor of the official drug is between 10 – 14 for seeds and 20 for husk. *Plantago lanceolata,* with its low mucilage content has a swelling factor around 4.75 and is therefore a potential adulterant. The seeds are yellowish brown in colour, oblong, elliptical and measure 2 to 3 mm in length and 0.7 to 1 mm in width.

JALAP

Source: Jalap consists of dried tuberous roots or tubercles of *Ipomoea purga* Hayane (Fam. Convolvulaceae).

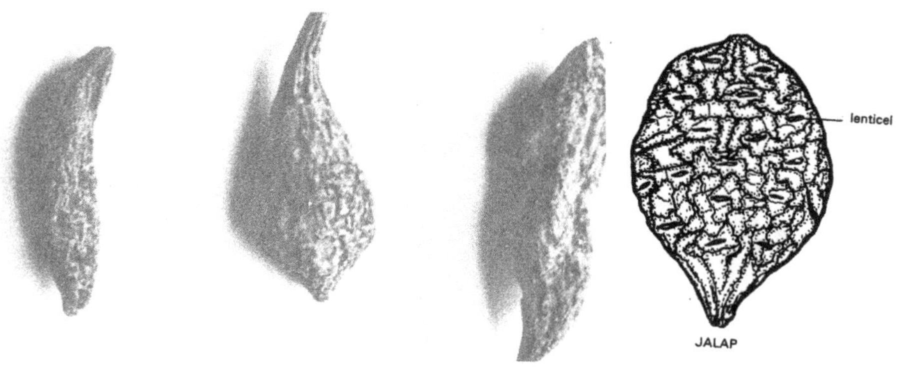

Synonyms and Regional Names: Mexican Jalap, Ben. (Hin.) Mirchai; Guj. Garayo.

Morphology: Form – irregularly oblong, napiform or fusiform; Colour – dark brown; Size – 3 to 15 cm(l), 3 – 8 cm (maximum diameter); Surface – longitudinal wrinkles with transverse lenticels; Odour – slight and smokey; Taste – first sweet and then acrid.

Active Constituents
RESINS – Glycosidal resin (8 – 20%), Convolvulin, Jalapin.

Therapeutical and Pharmaceutical Use: A Hydrogogue cathartic (a drug which discharges watery fluid).

JATAMANSI

Source: Jatamansi consists of the dried rhizomes and roots of *Nardostachys jatamansi* DC. (Fam. Valerianaceae).

Synonym and Regional Name: Jatamansi.

Morphology: Colour – dark grey, while internally reddish brown; Form – short, thick (size of a little finger), covered by group of brown fibres (the fibres are due to accumulation of the skeleton of leaves which get matted). Odour – aromatic like that of Valerian; Taste – bitter and aromatic.

Active Constituents
VOLATILE OIL (0.3 to 0.4%) – Sesquiterpenes – Valeranone

Therapeutical and Pharmaceutical Uses
1. Substitute for Valerian.
2. A good plant sedative.
3. In spasmodic attacks of hysteria, palpitation of heart etc.

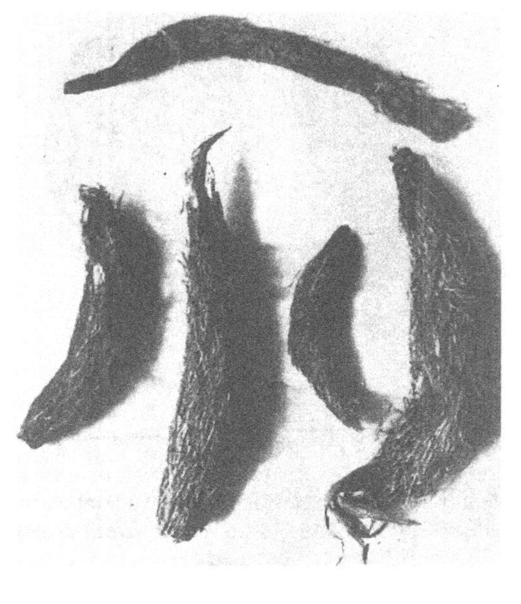
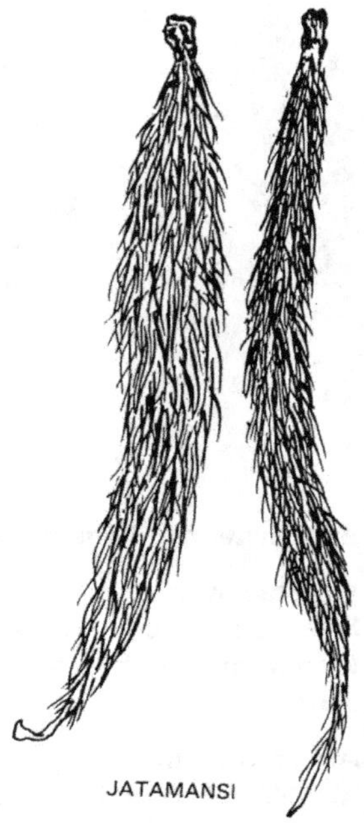

KALADANA

Source: Kaladana consists of the dried ripe seeds of *Ipomoea hederacea* Jacq.(Fam.

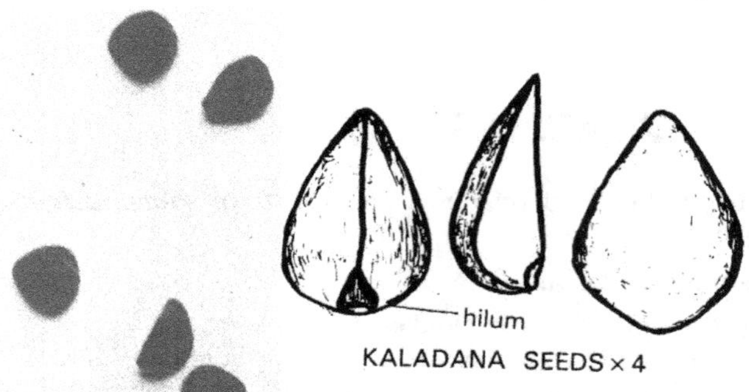

Synonyms and Regional Names
Pharbitis seeds
Ben. Nilkalmi
Guj. Kaladana
Hin. Mirhai
Kan. Gouribija
Mar. Milpushpi
Tam. Jirkivirai
Tel. Kolli vittulu

Morphology: Shape – roughly triangular, with two flat faces; Colour – dark black; Size – 5.5 mm(l) and 3.7 mm(w); Surface – hilum prominent situated at the base of the broad end; Odour – none and Taste – acrid.

Active Constituents
GLYCOSIDES – resin glycosides (8%)
FIXED OIL, SAPONINS

Therapeutical and Pharmaceutical Use: Hydrogogue purgative (discharging watery fluid).

KALMEGH

Source: Kalmegh consists of the dried or fresh entire aerial portion of the plant *Andrographis paniculata* Nees (Fam. Acanthaceae).

Synonyms and Regional Name: Andrographis, Ben. Kalmegh, Guj. Kariyatu, Hin. Kiryet, Kan. Nelabevu, Mal. Nelavepu, Mar. Olikirayet, San. Bhunimba Kirata, Tam. Nilavembu, Shirat kuchi, Tel. Nelavemu.

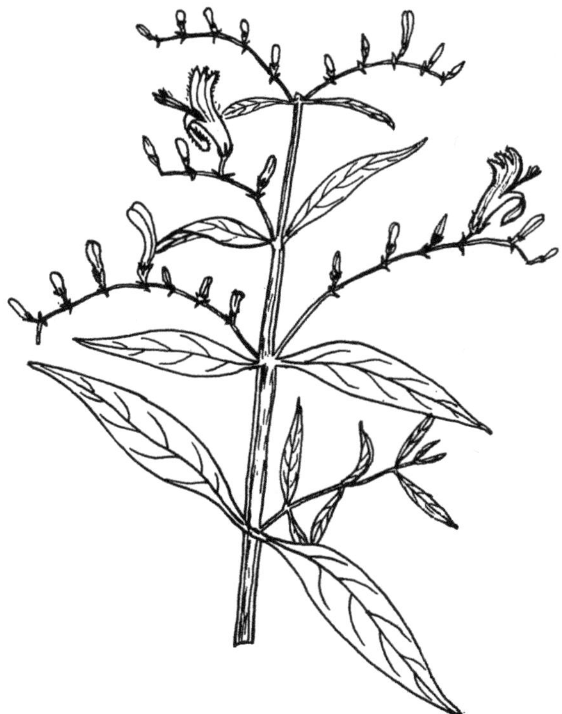

Morphology: Stem: Form – quadrangular with longitudinal furrows and wings and enlarged at nodes; Colour – dark green, size – about 1 m(h) and 2 – 6 mm(d). Leaves-arrangement-opposite decussate, shape-lanceolate, Colour-green, Size-upto 8 cm(l) and 2.5 cm(b); Surface – glabrous, margin-entire or slightly undulate, apex-acuminate with tapering base, pinnate venation and with very short petiole. Flowers – small, solitary, bilabiate, with light pink coloured corolla, Fruit-capsule, linear, oblong and acute at either ends. Seeds – numerous; Odour – none, Taste – intensely bitter.

FLOWERING TOP OF KALMEGH

Active Constituents
BITTER PRINCIPLES – Andrographolides (crystalline non-glycosidic principles).
FLAVONOIDS – Echidinin – Wightin – Serpyllin.

Therapeutical and Pharmaceutical Uses
1. As a bitter tonic and stomachic.
2. To relieve griping, irregular stools and loss of appetite in case of infants.
3. Febrifuge, alterative and anthelmintic.
4. In general debility, dysentery and certain forms of dyspepsia.
5. Reported to heal peptic ulcer.

KAOLIN

Source: Kaolin or hydrated aluminium silicate is a pure variety of clay, powdered and freed from gritty particles and other impurities.

Synonyms and Regional Names: China clay, Porcelain clay, Ben. Girimati, Hin. Chikminati, San. Gairika, Krishnamrittika.

Chemical Constituents: ALUMINIUM SILICATE and in traces magnesium, calcium and iron.

Therapeutical and Pharmaecutical Uses

1. Light Kaolin is used in cases of some gastric and intestinal affection.
2. Heavy Kaolin is used as a Pharmaceutical aid in Poultices and as pill excipients.

KAPUR KACHRI

Source: Kapur Kachri consists of the rhizomes and roots of *Hedychium spicatum* Ham. ex. Smith (Fam. Zingiberaceae).

Synonyms and Regional Names: Ben. Gandha Shaty, Hin. Sit-ruti, Kapur-Kachri, Sathi, Mar. Kapur Kachri, San. Kapura Kachali, Tam. Shimai kich-chilik, Kishangu.

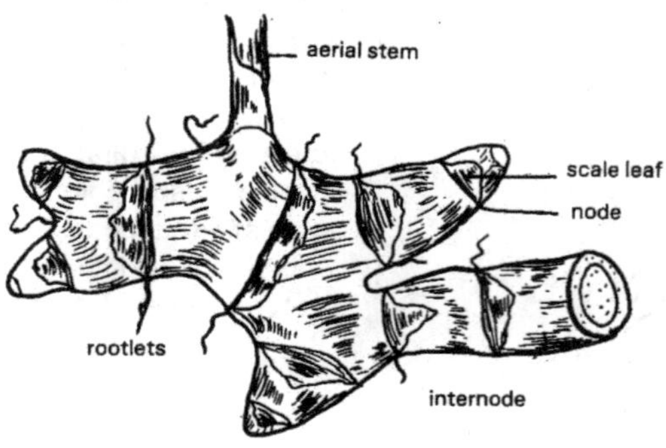

Morphology: Form – commercial samples appear in the form of slices; Size – upto 1.25 cm(d), upto 6 mm(t), Colour – reddish brown; Surface – rough and with rootlets attached here and there; Fracture – short, Fractured surface – white and starchy; Odour – aromatic; Taste – camphoraceous and bitter.

Active Constituents: ESSENTIAL OIL (4%)
— Cineole, Limonene, γ–terenene, β–phellandrene, p–cymene, Linalool, β–terpineol, β–caryophyllene, ethyl-p-methoxy cinnamate, –ethyl cinnamate, d–sabinene.
DITERPENE – a furanoid diterpene-7-hydroxy hedychinone.

Therapeutical and Pharmaceutical Uses: 1. Insect repellant, 2. Stomachic, carminative, tonic and stimulant, 3. Expectorant, 4. Emmenagogue, 5. In liver complaints, 6. Mild tranquillizer, 7. Anti-inflammatory, 8. Anthelminitic, 9. In the treatment of pulmonary eosinophilia.

KESAR

Source: Kesar is the dried stigma of *Crocus sativus* L. (Fam. Iridaceae).

Synonyms and Regional Name: Crocus, Saffron, Ben. Zafran, Guj. Mar. Keshar, Hin. Kesar, Zafran, Kan. Kesari, San. Kumkuma, Tam. Kungumapu, Tel. Kukumpuva.

Morphology: Stigmas: Colour—dark red to pale reddish brown, Shape—long, cornucopia shape, 3 in number, attached to the tip of the style or free, Size—about 2.5 cm(l); Margin—dentate or fimbriate; Styles—10 mm(l), cylindrical, solid, yellowish brown to yellowish orange; Odour – strong and characteristically aromatic; Taste – aromatic and bitter.

Active Constituents: CAROTENOIDS

Crocin, a coloured glycoside (Crocin on hydrolysis yields Crocetin + gentiobiose) – picrocrocin, a colourless bitter monoterpenoid glycoside (Safranol + glucose). Safranol is responsible for the characteristic and pleasant odour.

VOLATILE OIL (0.4 to 1.3%) – terpenes, terpene alcohols and esters.

Therapeutical and Pharmaceutical Uses

1. Flavouring and Colouring agent.
2. Taste corrector.
3. Stomachic and Antispasmodic.
4. Stimulant and Aphrodisiac.
5. Nerve sedative.
6. Emmenagogue (promotes the menstrual flow).

Chemical Test: When Kesar is placed in H_2SO_4 a deep blue colour is seen.

KOKUM BUTTER

Source: Kokum Butter is an edible fat (39%) obtained by expression from the seeds of *Garcinia indica* Choisy (Fam. Guttiferae).

Synonyms and Regional Names: Brindolia tallow, Mangosteen oil; Guj. Hin. Kokam; Mar. Amsol; Bhirand; Katambi, Kokam, Ratamba; Kan. Murgala; Tam. Murgal.

Nature: Colour—greyish white to white; Form – market samples consist of egg shaped lumps or cakes with a greasy feel and bland oily taste.

Active Constituents: LIPIDS-TRIGLYCERIDES

FATTY ACIDS — rich in combined stearic and oleic acids-stearic (56.4%), oleic (39.4%), palmitic (2.5%) and linoleic (1.7%).

Therapeutical and Pharmaceutical Uses

1. Nutritive, demulcent, astringent and emollient (soothing agent).
2. As a pharmaceutical aid in preparation of ointments and suppositories etc.

KURCHI

Source: Kurchi consists of the dried stem bark of *Holarrhena antidysenterica* Wall. (Fam. Apocynaceae) collected from plants which are 8 to 12 years old, freed from attached wood and peeled into small pieces. It contains not less than 2.0% of the total alkaloids of Kurchi.

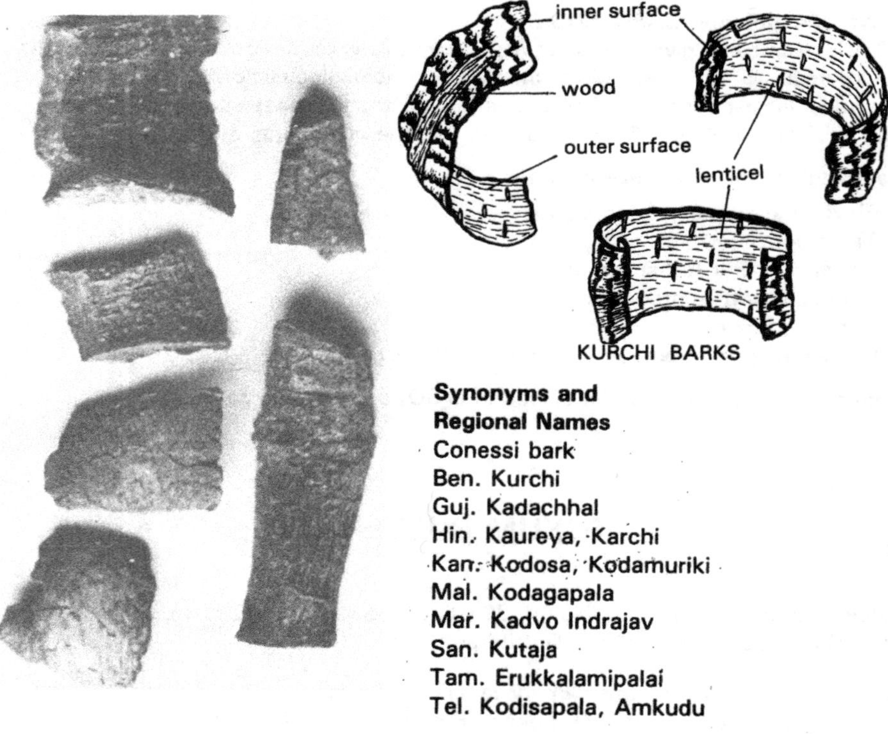

Synonyms and Regional Names

Conessi bark
Ben. Kurchi
Guj. Kadachhal
Hin. Kaureya, Karchi
Kan. Kodosa, Kodamuriki
Mal. Kodagapala
Mar. Kadvo Indrajav
San. Kutaja
Tam. Erukkalamipalai
Tel. Kodisapala, Amkudu

Morphology: Condition — dry; Shape — longitudinally recurved pieces; Colour — buff to light brown; Size — variable; Outer surface — transverse lenticels are prominent so also fine longitudinal wrinkles; Inner surface — brownish, rough and with irregular transverse cracks. Light yellow wood may be seen attached occasionally; Fracture – short and granular; Odour – none and Taste – bitter.

Active Constituents

ALKALOIDS – Steroidal alkaloids (2 – 4%)

Conessine (30%), Norconessine, Isoconessine, Kurchicine, Holarrhimine and Holarrhenine.

Therapeutical and Pharmaceutical Uses

1. In the treatment of dysentery (used both in acute and chronic dysentery).
2. Astringent and Tonic.
3. As an antiperiodic (used in periodic recurrence like Malaria).
4. In the synthesis of steroid hormones.
5. Kurchi is used in 59 drug preparations (Kapoor & Mitra).

LANOLIN

Source: Lanolin is obtained by purifying fat like substances from the wool of the sheep *Ovis aries* L. (Fam. Bovidae). The water content should be between 25 – 30% hence the name hydrous wool fat.

Nature: Colour – yellowish white; Consistency – ointment like; Odour – slight but characteristic.

Chemical Composition: LIPIDS

— Fats – Cholesterol, isocholesterol, esters of fatty acids like lanopalmitic, lanoceric, carnaubic, oleic, myristic etc.

Therapeutical and Pharmaceutical Uses

1. Water absorbable ointment base.
2. Emollient base for creams, ointments and cosmetics.

Note: Wool Fat or Anhydrous Lanolin is Lanolin containing not more than 0.25% of water.

Chemical Test: The test is based on the presence of cholesterol. 0.5 g of Lanolin is dissolved in 5 ml of chloroform. Addition of 1 ml acetic anhydride and 2 drops of H_2SO_4 results in a deep green colour.

LEHSUN

Source: Lehsun is the fresh compound bulb of *Allium sativum* Linn. (Fam. Liliaceae).

Synonyms and Regional Names: Garlic,Ben. Rasun; Guj. Lasun; Hin. Lehsun; Kan. Belluli; Mar. Lasun; Tam. Vallaippundu; Mal. Tel. Velluli.

Morphology: Type – Sub-globular compound bulb with several cloves, enclosed in a silky white or pinkish papery envelope of the skin. The cloves are attached to a flat, circular, hard axis with numerous thin wiry roots from its underside and short-cylindrical outgrowths from the upper surface. Each clove is ovoid, surrounded by two

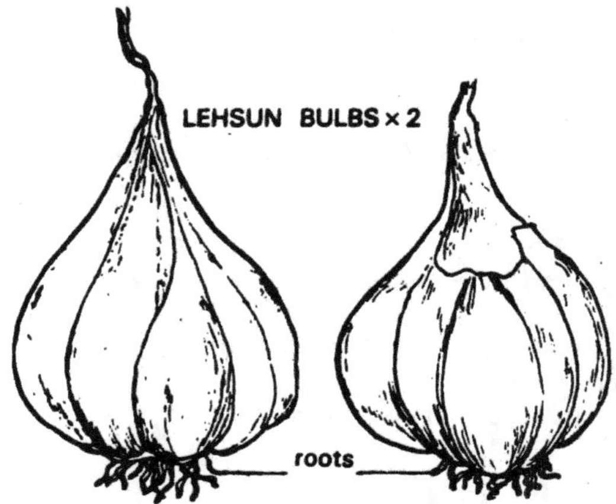

papery scale leaves, the outer one whitish and loose, the inner one pink and adherent, but easily separable from the solid portion of the clove; the papery scale leaves enclose two whitish, fleshy scales, the inner one thinner and smaller than the outer. The foliage leaves present in the centre are yellowish green; Odour — strongly alliaceous and Taste — strongly pungent and alliaceous.

Active Constituents: ESSENTIAL OIL (0.1 to 0.3%)
— Alliin, a sulphur containing amino acid
— Allicin — Allyl sulphide
— Polysulphides responsible for the unpleasant smell of the oil.

Therapeutical and Pharmaceutical Uses

1. Flavouring agent.
2. Anti-bacterial.
3. In cases of hypertension and atherosclerosis (thickening of arterial wall).
4. In the treatment of malignant tumours.
5. Carminative, gastric stimulant and aids in digestion and absorption of food.
6. Oil of garlic is used as an insecticide.

LEMONGRASS OIL

Source: Lemongrass Oil is the volatile oil obtained by steam distillation from the leaves of *Cymbopogon citratus* (DC) Stapf. (Fam. Graminae).

Synonyms and Regional Names: Indian Oil of Verbena, Indian Melissa Oil; Ben. Gandhbenar; Tel. Hin. Gandhbina ka tel; Mar. Hirvacha tel.

Nature: Colour — dark yellow to brownish red; Odour — strong and characteristic.

Chemical Constituents

— Citral (65 to 86%) — geraniol, myrcin (12 – 20%) — methyl heptenone.
— dipentene — citronellal — linalool, α-terpineol.

Therapeutical and Pharmaceutical Uses

1. In the commercial production of Citral.
2. In the soap industry.
3. As a taste corrector in liquor industry.

LEMON PEEL

Source: Lemon Peel is the outer part of the ripe or nearly ripe fruit of *Citrus limon* L. Burm. (Fam. Rutaceae). The fruit is gathered when green and nearly ripe.

Synonyms and Regional Names: Lemon peel; Ben. Neboo;Hin. Kambira-ka-chilka; Kan. Nimbe-sippe; Mal. Cherunaranga-tholi; Mar. Limbacha-sal; San. Jambira; Tam. Elumichhampalam; Tel. Nimmapandu.

Morphology: Fresh pieces: Colour – greenish yellow on the outer surface; Nature – smooth, oily, glossy and more or less pitted; Small amount of the white spongy pericarp is seen on the inner surface; Odour – sweet and aromatic· Taste – bitter.

Active Constituents

VOLATILE OIL (2 – 5%) — Aldehydes like Citral and Citronellal
— Terpenes like Limonene (90%) etc.

FLAVONOIDS – Neohesperidin and Naringin
VITAMIN C

Therapeutical and Pharmaceutical Uses

1. Flavouring agent.
2. Pharmaceutical aid.

LICORICE

Source: Licorice consists of the dried, peeled or unpeeled, root and stolon of *Glycyrrhiza glabra* L. (Fam. Leguminosae) and other species of *Glycyrrhiza*.

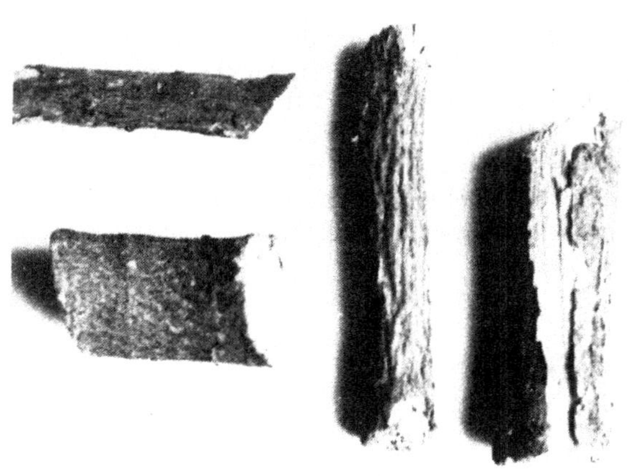

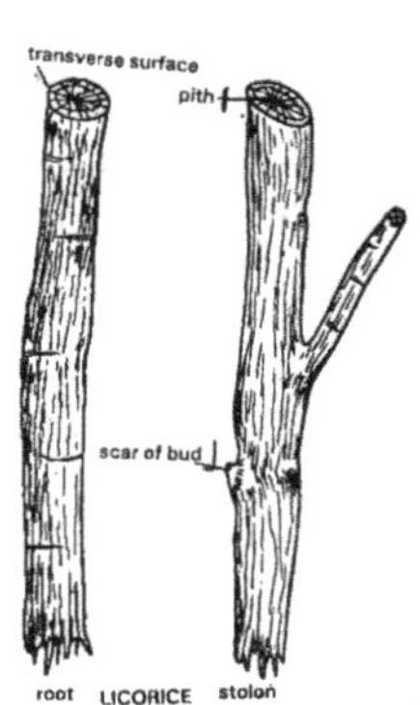

Synonyms and Regional Names: Glycyrrhizae Radix, Liquorice root; Ben. Jasthimadhu; Guj. Jethimadha; Hin. Jetimadhu, Mulethi; Kan. Jhesta Madhu; Mal. Yera Himadhuram; Mar. Jashtimadh; San. Yasthimadhu; Tam. Atimadhuram; Tel. Atimadhuramu.

Morphology: Condition – dry, occurs in the peeled or unpeeled forms; Shape – cylindrical; Surface (outer) – yellowish brown with longitudinal wrinkles (unpeeled); Peeled ones are yellow coloured with fine longitudinal ridges. In case of stolons, scars of buds can be seen. Fracture – coarsely fibrous in the bark region and splintery in the wood; Fractured surface shows long fibres projecting outwards. In stolons pith may be seen in the transverse surface; Odour – characteristic and Taste – sweet.

Active Constituents

GLYCOSIDES – Saponin glycoside – 18 β Glycyrrhizin (3 – 9%)
$\qquad\qquad\qquad$ 18 β Glycyrrhetic acid (aglycone)
$\qquad\qquad$ Flavonoids – Liquiritin – Liquiritigenin
$\qquad\qquad\qquad\qquad$ – Isoliquiritin – Isoliquiritigenin
$\qquad\qquad$ Coumarin derivatives – Herniarin – Umbelliferone

Chemical test: Licorice on treatment with sulphuric acid gives yellow colour due to the conversion of flavonoid glycoside liquiritin to chalcone glycoside isoliquiritin.

Therapeutical and Pharmaceutical Uses

1. Demulcent (soothing) and expectorant (promotes the removal of catarrhal matter and phlegm from the bronchial tubes).
2. Laxative in combination with other drugs.
3. As an anti-inflammatory agent in dermatological practice (in peptic ulcer).
4. Spasmolytic agent (arrests involuntary muscular contraction).
5. To mask the bitter taste.
6. Licorice is used in 141 drug preparations (Kapoor & Mitra).

Substitutes and Adulterants: Manchurian Licorice is obtained from *Glycyrrhiza uralensis.* Colour is chocolate brown and cork exfoliating. Anatomically also it shows peculiarities based on which one can distinguish. The medullary rays are curved and presence of lacunae can be seen in the wood. Being a substitute it does contain glycyrrhizin the active principle but very little of free sugars. The common adulterant is wild licorice also called Indian Licorice, derived from the roots of *Abrus precatorius* (Leguminosae). The roots are very toxic due to an alkaloid abrine and therefore should not be used in place of licorice. The roots possess a peculiar disagreeable odour and bitter acrid flavour leaving faintly sweet after taste. Microscopically the adulterant is characterized by stone cells.

LINSEED

Source: Linseed is the dried ripe seed of *Linum usitatissimum* L. (Fam. Linaceae). It contains not less that 25% of fixed oil.

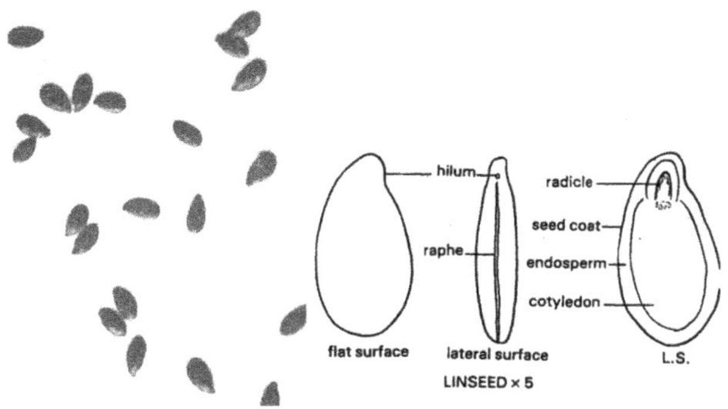

Synonyms and Regional Names
Flax seed
Ben. Masina
Guj. Alasi
Hin. Alsi
Kan. Atasi bija, Agashi
Mal. Cerucanam vithu
Mar. Javas
San. Atasi bija
Tam. Alishivirai
Tel. Avisi vettu

Morphology: Shape—ovoid or oblong-lanceolate, flattened obliquely pointed to one end; Size—4–6 mm(l) 2–3 mm(w); Colour—brown; Surface—smooth and shining and minutely pitted; hilum and micropyle in a slight depression just below the pointed end. From the hilum the raphe which is yellowish in colour runs to the other end; Odourless and mucilaginous and oily in taste.

Active Constituents: FIXED OIL (30–40%)

MUCILAGE (6%)   —   yielding on hydrolysis→galactose (8–12%)—arabinose (9–12%)—rhamnose (13–29%)—xylose (25–27%) —galacturonic acid—mannuronic acid (30%)

PROTEIN (25%)

GLYCOSIDE   —   Cyanogenetic glycosides—Linamarin (1–5%)
—Lotaustralin

Therapeutical and Pharmaceutical Uses
1. Externally as a poultice.
2. Internally as Demulcent (soothing).
3. Laxative and in cases of Hemorrhoids.
4. To extract 'linseed oil'.

LOBELIA

Source: Lobelia consists of dried aerial parts of *Lobelia nicotianaefolia* Heyne (Fam. Lobeliaceae), collected in October and November and dried in shade. It contains not less than 0.55% of total alkaloids calculated as lobeline.

Synonyms and Regional Names: Wild tobacco Ben. Bantamaku, Badanal, Guj. Nali, Hin. Nala, Narasala, Mal. Kattupukaila, Mar. Devnala, San. Bibhishana, Devnala, Tam. Kattuppugaiyilai, Tel. Adavipogaku.

Morphology: Stems: Form—rounded, channelled, usually branched at the top; Colour—green with a purplish-tint; Surface—somewhat pubescent, Leaves—alternate, subsessile, obovate lanceolate, acute, finely serrulate; Upper

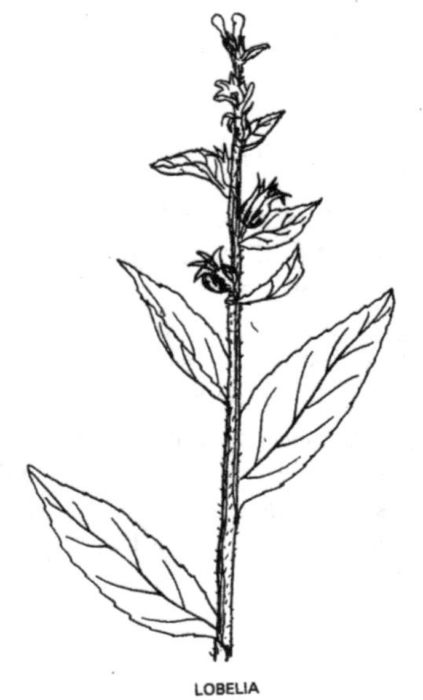

LOBELIA

surface is glabrous, whereas glabrous to pubescent beneath; Fruit-longitudinally ribbed, subglobose, inflated capsule; Seeds-small, ellipsoidal, compressed, coarsely reticulate; Odourless but with extremely acrid and irritating taste.

Active Constituents: ALKALOIDS.
Piperidine type – Lobeline – isolobinine

Therapeutical and Pharmaceutical Uses:
1. Used in spasmodic asthma and chronic bronchitis. 2. The physiological action is similar to that of nicotine. 3. In cases of resuscitation (restoration to life of one apparently dead).

MALE FERN

Source: Male Fern consists of rhizomes and frond bases of *Dryopteris filix-mas* Linn. (Schott.) containing not less than 1.5% of filicin, (Fam. Aspidiaceae). The drug is collected late in autumn, divested of roots and dead portions, and carefully dried, retaining their internal green colour.

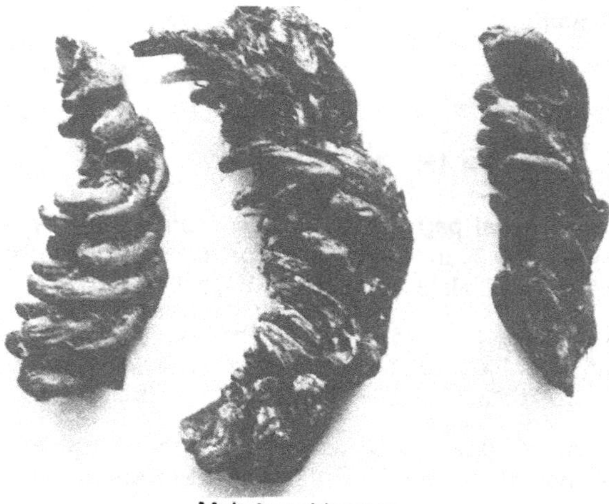

Male fern rhizomes

Synonyms
Aspidium
Dryopteris, filix-mas

Morphology
Shape – irregular;
Colour – dark brown (external), yellowish green (internal), Size – 7 – 25 cm(l), 2 – 4 cm(d); Surface – completely covered with hard dark brown to black curved leaf bases bearing numerous membranous ramenta; Fracture – short, fractured surface – earthy brown; Odourless,

Taste – in the beginning sweetish and astringent, later bitter and nauseous.

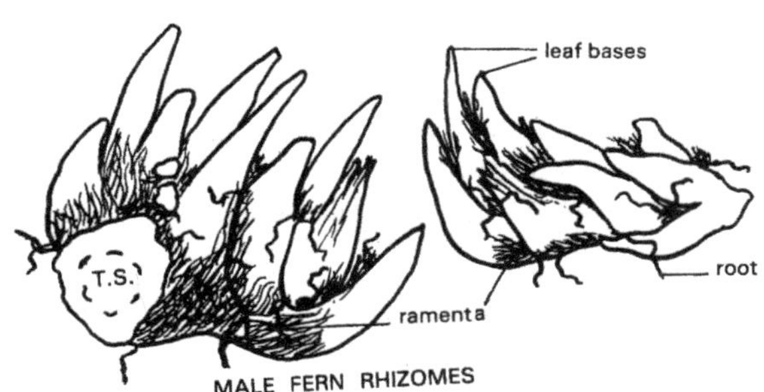

Active Constituents:
OLEORESINS (6.5 – 15%)
Phloroglucinol derivatives
– aspidinol, albaspidine,
filicic acid (filicin).

Therapeutical and Pharmaceutical Use: Anthelmintic (a drug which kills the intestinal worms) – Taenicide.

Field Test: The cut surface retains greenish tinge for long time even after drying.

Substitutes and adulterants: Both Lady Fern (*Athyrium filix-foemina*) and Shield Fern (*Dryopteris spinulosa*) are often known to occur along with the official drug. In case of Lady Fern, margin of the ramenta is entire and the steles in the frond bases are two in number and are dumb-bell shaped. The margins of the ramenta in case of shield fern possess small glands.

MENTHA OIL

Source: Mentha Oil is the volatile oil distilled with steam from fresh aerial parts of various species of *Mentha* like *M. piperita* L. (Fam. Labiatae). It contains not less than 50% of total menthol.

Synonyms: Peppermint oil, Peppermint.

Nature: Colourless or pale yellow liquid; Odour – strong and penetrating; Taste – pungent and sensation of cool feeling when air is drawn into the mouth.

Active Constituents
VOLATILE OIL — Menthol (50%) – Menthone (10 – 30%)
— Piperitone – Menthylester – Menthofuran (5 – 10%).

Therapeutical and Pharmaceutical Uses

1. Carminative.
2. Spasmolytic.
3. Cholagogue.
4. Mild antidiarrhoetic.
5. In tooth paste preparations as a taste corrector.
6. Aromatic stimulant – stimulates the nerve endings which are sensitive to cold and gives a cool feeling.

MUSTARD

Source: Black or brown mustard is the dried ripe seeds of *Brassica nigra* Koch or *B. juncea* (Fam. Cruciferae) and their varieties.

Synonyms and Regional Names: Ben. Sarisha; Guj. Rai; Hin. Rai; Kalee Sarson; Kan. Sasave; San. Asuri, bimbata; Tam. Kadugo; Tel. Avalu.

Morphology: Shape – spherical to globular; Size – 1.5 mm(d); Colour – dark reddish brown externally and yellow internally; Surface – minutely pitted, odourless; Taste – to begin with mild only, weakly acidic and finally strongly pungent.

Active Constituents

FIXED OIL (25 to 30%) — glycerides of following unsaturated fatty acids (90%)
— oleic acid, linoleic acid and linolinic acid.
— Glycerides of saturated fatty acids (10%)

VOLATILE OIL (0.7 to 1.3%) — is obtained on hydrolysing the isothiocyanate (Allyl isothiocyanate) glycoside – Sinigrin (1 – 1.2%), with the enzyme myrosin

Proteins, mucilage etc. (30%)

Therapeutical and Pharmaceutical Uses

1. Expressed oil has mild rubefacient properties and is used in liniments and plasters.   2. Used as condiment.   3. Emetic when taken in large doses.

MYROBALAN

Source: Myrobalan consists of the dried fruits of *Terminalia chebula* Retz (Fam. Combretaceae) and are available in two forms; the semi-mature fruits and young fruits of smaller size.

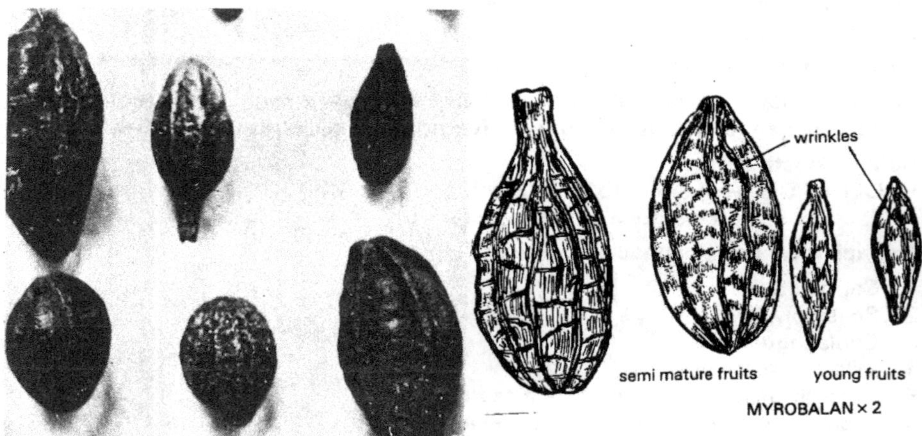

Synonyms and Regional Names: Ben. Haritaki; Guj. Hirdo; Hin. Harara; Kan. Aralaikai; Male Divya; Mar. Hirda; San. Haritaki; Tam. Kadukki; Tel. Karikaki.

Morphology: Semi-mature fruits; Colour – yellowish brown; Shape – ovoid Size – 20-35 mm(l) 13 – 25 mm(w); Surface – wrinkled longitudinally, hard and stony; Seed colour – light yellow; Size — 15 – 25 mm(l) and the thick pulp is non-adherent to the seed. Odourless and Taste – astringent and somewhat sweetish.

86

Young Fruits; Colour – deep brown to black; Shape – elongated, ovoid both sides tapering; Size – smaller in size than semi-mature fruits; Surface – hard with longitudinal ribs and wrinkles; Odourless and Taste – astringent and bitter.

Active Constituents

TANNINS (30%) — pyrogallol type – chebulagic acid (ellagi tannins)

     — chebulinic acid, chebulic acid; ellagic acid.

     — gallic acid etc.

Oleoresins, carbohydrates, a non-nitrogenous principle-chebulin and some purgative principles.

Therapeutical and Pharmaceutical Uses

1. As an external applicant to chronic ulcers and wounds.
2. As a gargle in stomatitis.
3. Laxative. ·
4. External application relieves headache.
5. Myrobalan as an ingredient of "Triphala" is used in 219 drug preparations (Kapoor & Mitra).

MYRRH

Source: Myrrh is the oleo-gum-resin obtained by incision from the stem of *Commiphora molmol* Engler (Fam. Burseraceae).

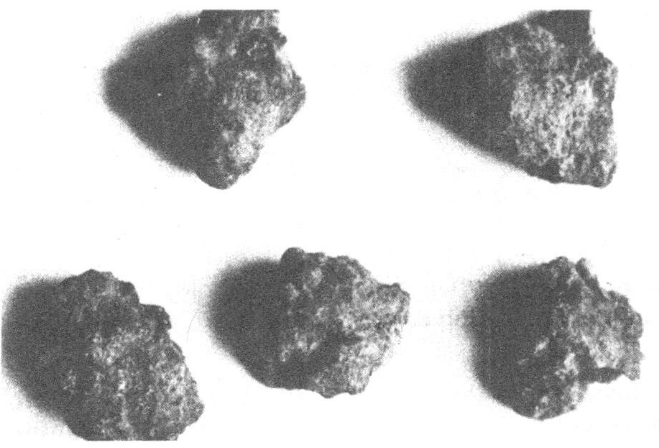

Synonyms and Regional Names

Myrrha, Arabian or Somali Myrrh

Ben. Gandharash

Guj. Hirabol

Hin. Bol

Kan. Bola

Mar. Hirabol

San. Vola, Rasagandha, Saindhava

Tam. Vellaippapolam

Tel. Balintrapolum

Morphology: Form – irregular rounded tears or lumps of agglutinated tears; Colour – reddish yellow or reddish brown; Size – variable; Surface – rough, covered with fine yellow powder; Fracture – brittle, fractured surface brown, shining, oily and with whitish marks; Odour – aromatic; Taste – bitter.

Active Constituents: VOLATILE OIL (2.5 – 8%)

 phenol-eugenol – cuminic aldehyde, – α pinene – limonene and sesquiterpenes

RESIN (25 – 40%) – Resin acids like, α-β-γ-commiphoric acids

GUMS (60%) – yield on hydrolysis arabinose, galactose, 4-0-methyl glucuronic acid and aldobiuronic acid.

Therapeutical and Pharmaceutical Uses: 1. Antiseptic 2. Stimulant 3. Used in mouth wash and tooth paste 4. In perfume industry.

Chemical Tests

1. A yellowish brown emulsion is obtained when myrrh is triturated with water.
2. An ethereal solution of the drug attains reddish colour when treated with Br_2 vapours whereas purple colour when moistened with nitric acid. These two distinguishing tests are not answered by Bdellium (a species of *Commiphora*).

NUTMEG

Source: Nutmeg consists the dried kernels of the seeds of *Myristica fragrans* Houtt. (Fam. Myristicaceae). It contains not less than 5% v/w. of volatile oil.

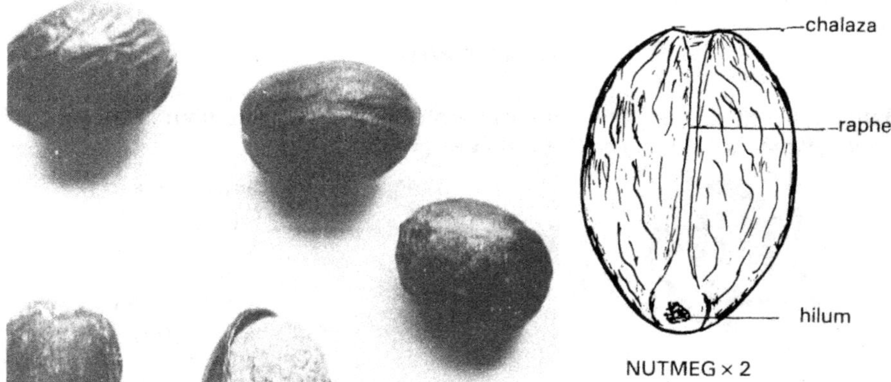

Synonyms and Regional Names: Ben. Jayphal; Guj., Hin. Mar. Jayaphal; Kan. Jaikai; Mal. Jatika; San. Jatiphalam. Jaiphala, Rajika; Tam. Jadikkay; Tel. Jajikaya.

Morphology: Shape – ovoid depending on the variety either broad or elongated; Colour – light brown to greyish brown; Size – 2 – 3 cm(l) and 1.5 – 2 cm(b); Surface – shows a network of shallow reticulate grooves and is marked with numerous small dark brown points and lines; Odour – aromatic and characteristic; Taste – aromatic and bitter.

Active Constituents

VOLATILE OIL (4 – 16%) – Myristicin (4 – 8%), pinene, sabinene, camphene, Safrole, Eugenol, Methyl eugenol, isoeugenol, methyl isoeugenol, methoxy eugenol.

FIXED OIL (25 – 30%), SAPONIN etc.

Therapeutical and Pharmaceutical Uses
1. Flavouring agent   2. Carminative (relieves excessive gas collected in the stomach)   3. Digestive – increases the appetite   4. Abortifacient (an agent that promotes abortion).

NUX VOMICA

Source: Nux Vomica consists of the dried, ripe seeds of *Strychnos nux-vomica* L. (Fam. Loganiaceae). It contains not less than 1.2% of Strychnine.

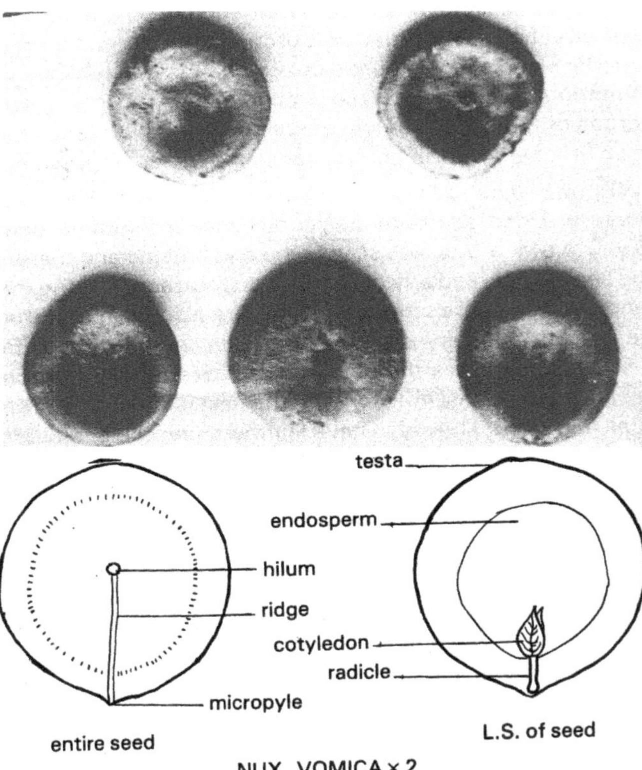

Synonyms and Regional Names
Poison nut tree
Ben. Kuchila
Guj. Zer kachuro
Kan. Kasarkana
Mal. Kanjiram
Mar. Kajra
San. Vishamushti
Tam. Yettimaram
Tel. Mushtimanu

Morphology: Size – 10 – 30 mm(d) and 4 to 6 mm(t); Shape – disc shaped, sometimes flat, little depressed on one side and arched on the other, sometimes irregularly bent. Margin more or less rounded; O. Surface – ash grey or greyish grey covered with numerous closely appressed silky hairs, radiating from the centre. Hilum is present in the centre of one of the flat surfaces. Micropyle is seen as a small projecting point on the margin. Hilum and micropyle are connected by a ridge; L.S. – Embryo is seen at the micropylar end with a cylindrical radicle and two cordate cotyledons. Endosperm is translucent, greyish in colour and with a white embryo; Odour – none and Taste–very bitter.

Active Constituents

ALKALOIDS (2.5 to 5%) – Indole type – Strychnine – Brucine
GLYCOSIDE – Monoterpene glycoside – Loganin
FIXED OIL (2 to 4%)

Therapeutical and Pharmaceutical Uses

Strychnine is therapeutically active whereas Brucine is less active or inactive.
1. Spinalcord stimulant.   2. In cases of neurasthenia (excessive fatigue of neurotic origin).   3. As a circulatory stimulant   4. Nerve and sex tonic.   5. Bitter stomachic (strengthening of stomach and promoting its action).

Chemical Tests

Distinguishing test for Strychnine and Brucine: To the residue from an extract of the drug, on addition of 2 drops of sulphovanadic acid formation of purple red colour indicates the presence of strychnine. Addition of 2 drops of H_2SO_4 and a crystal of Pot dichromate to another sample, again purple colour changing to red indicates strychnine whereas formation of immediate red colour marks the presence of Brucine. Addition of 2 drops of HNO_3 to a sample of residue gives blood red colour showing the presence of Brucine. The blood red colour however disappears on adding to it a soln. of Stannous chloride.

Substitutes and Adulterants: Dried seeds of *Strychnos ignatii* (Ignatius beans) contain as much as 2.5 to 3% of the alkaloids strychnine and brucine and therefore used as a substitute. The seeds are irregularly ovoid with dull surfaces. Of the many surfaces, one is large and the others are small and flat. Here also as in the official drug, the trichomes are present but they are easily detachable and not lignified.

S. potatorum and *S. nux-blanda* are the common adulterants. *S. potatorum* commonly called as clearing nut does not contain the alkaloids and therefore not bitter. Seeds are small and thick. They also have lignified, unicellular epidermal trichomes which however can be distinguished from those of *S. nux-vomica.* Nuxblanda seeds are brighter and yellowish buff in colour and show a small ridge on the edge. Here again as the alkaloids are absent the seeds are not bitter.

OPIUM

Source: Opium is the air-dried latex obtained by incision from the unripe capsule of *Papaver somniferum* L. (Fam. Papaveraceae). It contains not less than 9.5% of morphine, calculated as anhydrous morphine.

Synonyms and Regional Names: White poppy, Ben. Posto-dheri; Guj. Afin; Hin. Afim; Kan. Afeemu; Mal. Apeem; Mar. Aphim; San. Aphiphena; Tam. Apin, Abhini; Tel. Nallamandu

Morphology: Form – cubical pieces weighing about 900 g wrapped in tissue paper Texture – hard and brittle to plastic; internally dark brown, smooth and homogeneous; Odour – strong and characteristic; Taste – bitter.

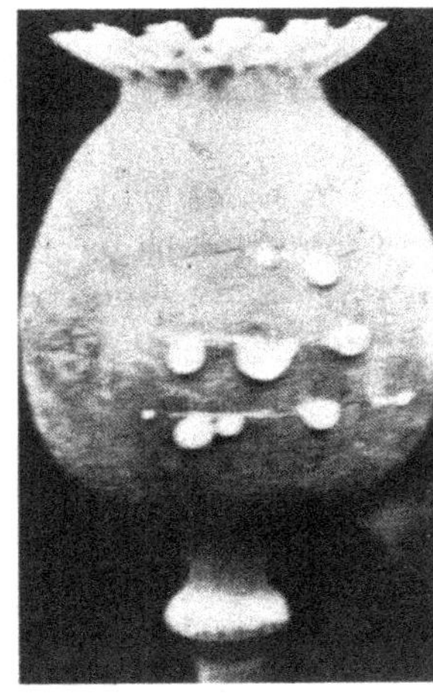 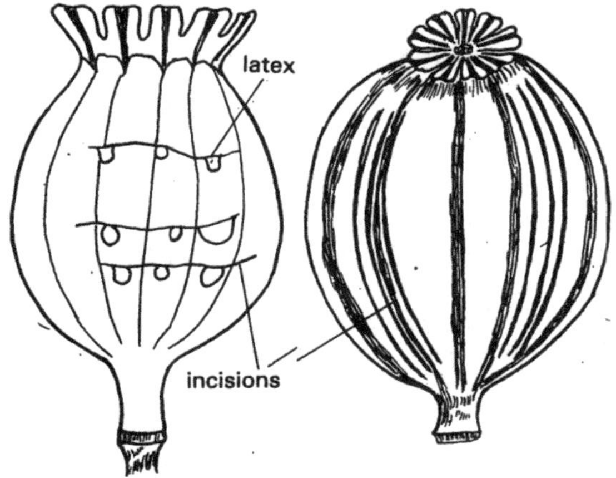

POPPY CAPSULES

Active Constituents

ALKALOIDS – Phenanthrene type – Morphine (10%), – Codeine (0.5%),
– Thebaine (0.2%)
– Benzylisoquinoline Type – Papaverine (1%), – Noscapine (6%),
– Narceine (0.3%) all in combination with Meconic acid (3 – 5%)

Therapeutical and Pharmaceutical Uses: 1. Analgesic (kills the pain). 2. Hypnotic (an agent that induces into a passive state or sleep) and Narcotic (a drug which produces sleep). 3. In case of cough and bronchitis. 4. In case of diarrhoea and dysentery. 5. In cases of Euphoria (a pleasant feeling of well-being with confidence and assurance).

Chemical Test: Since meconic acid is found only in Opium, a colour test based on this can be used to detect opium. Alkaloids of opium give a red colouration with ferric chloride soln. the colour being altered on addition of dil. HCl.

ORANGE PEEL

Source: Orange Peel is the dried outer part of the pericarp of the ripe or nearly ripe fruits of *Citrus chysocarpa* Lush. (*C. aurantium*) L. (Fam. Rutaceae).

Synonyms and Regional Names: Ben. Kamla; Guj. Musambi-Chal; Hin. Naranji-ka-chilka; Kan. Musambi sippe; Mal. Madhura-narakam, Narangathol; Mar. Santrachi sal; San. Nagaranga; Tam. Kitehli; Tel. Ganjanimma.

Active Constituents: VOLATILE OIL (2.5%) – Limonene – Citral – Citronellal – α Terpineol – Linalyl-and-Geranylacetate. |
VITAMIN C GLYCOSIDE – Flavonoid Glycosides (5 to 14%) – Hesperidin – Neohesperidin.

Therapeutical and Pharmaceutical Uses: 1. Flavouring agent 2. Bitter tonic 3. Source of Vitamin C and P.

PECTIN

Source: Pectin is a purified carbohydrate product obtained from the dilute acid extract of the inner portion of the rind of citrus fruits, apple fruits, etc. A number of fruits and their juices are rich in pectins (Lemon 2 to 5%). Purified pectin is obtained from these fruits by extracting with dilute acids.

Nature: Form – powder; Colour – yellowish white; Odourless and Taste – mucilaginous; Molecular weight – around 25,000 – 90,000; Solubility – soluble in water in the proportion of 1:20, the resulting soln. being viscous, colloidal and acidic whereas in a different proportion with water namely 1:9, it forms a stiff gel.

Chemistry: It is a linear polymer of galacturonic acid with 1:4 α linkage. Around 50% of the carboxyl groups are esterified with methanol. In some, the OH groups are partly acetylated.

Therapeutical and Pharmaceutical Uses: 1. In the treatment of diarrhoea and gastroenteritis. 2. In the treatment of wounds (2% sterile solution). 3. As a substitute for blood plasma. 4. In conjugation with Kaolin as an absorbant of intestine toxins. 5. To dampen and mask the taste. 6. As a thickening agent in the preparation of pills and tablets. 7. In the preparation of Heparinoids.

PHYSOSTIGMA

Source: Physostigma consists of the ripe seeds of *Physostigma venenosum* Balfour (Fam. Leguminosae) containing not less than 0.15% of alkaloids of Physostigma.

Morphology: Form – bean shaped; colour – dark brown; Size – 25 – 35 mm(l), 17 – 20 mm(w); Surface – rough near the groove which is brownish black in colour measuring 1 – 2 mm in diameter extending about half way around the edge containing the raphe and the micropyle. Drug is odourless but tastes sweetish and mealy.

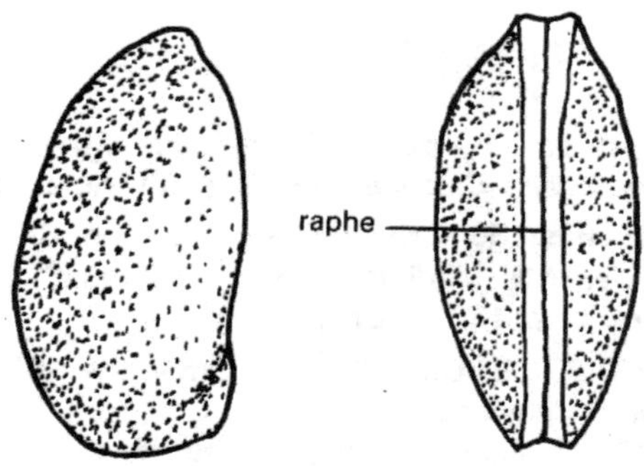

PHYSOSTIGMA SEEDS

Active Constituents: ALKALOIDS (0.1 – 0.4%) – Indole alkaloids.
– Physostigmine or Eserine (50% of the total alkaloids) – Geneserine.

Therapeutical and Pharmaceutical Uses: 1. In ophthalmology in the treatment of glaucoma.   2. A parasympathomimetic.

PICRORHIZA

Source: Picrorhiza consists of dried roots and rhizomes of *Picrorhiza kurroa* Royle ex Benth (Fam. Scrophulariaceae), cut in small pieces and freed from attached rootlets. It is called 'Indian Gentian' because of its bitter taste.

Synonyms and Regional Names: Ben. Katki; Guj. Kadu; Hin. Kutki, Kuru; Mal. Katukurohini; Mar. Kutaki; San. Katuka; Tam. Katuku-rogini; Tel. Katuku-roni.

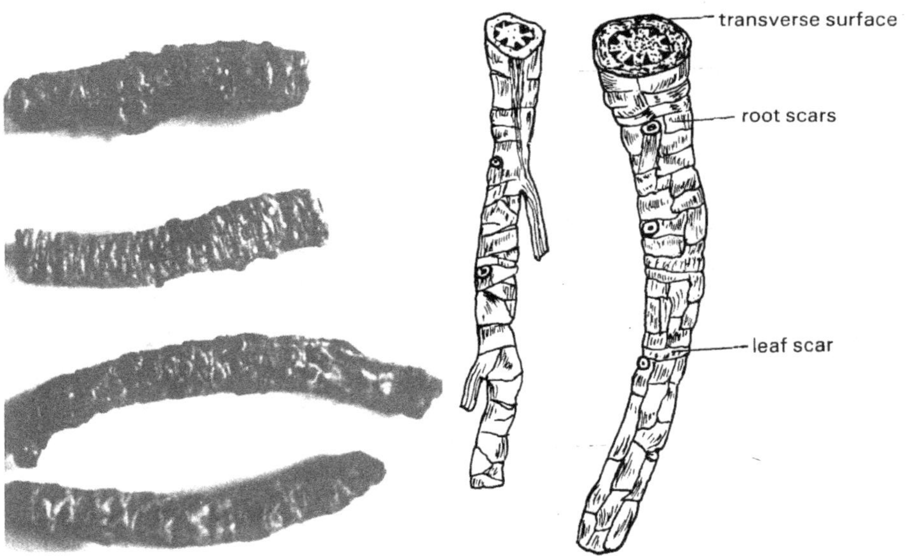

PICRORHIZA ROOTS

Morphology: Form – light, cylindrical, straight or slightly curved; Colour – greyish brown; Size – 2 to 5 cm(l), 4 to 8 mm(w); Surface – remains of dark brown and longitudinal wrinkles, aerial stems are often seen; so also a few small root scars and numerous semi-amplexicaul scale leaves are seen both on upper and lower surfaces; Odour – slightly unpleasant and very bitter to taste.

Active Constituents: GLYCOSIDES – Iridoid glycosides – Picrorhizin, Picroside A containing cinnamic acid – Kutkoside containing vanillic acid – Kurrin (0.5%), a nonbitter product – Kutkiol an alcohol – Kutkisterol a sterol and Cathartic acid.

Therapeutical and Pharmaceutical Uses:

1. Bitter tonic and used as a substitute for Gentian.
2. Febrifuge, Antiperiodic, Cholagogue (an agent which increases the flow of bile) and Stomachic.
3. Mild laxative.
4. In malaria associated with constipation.
5. Live ailment, jaundice and hepatitis.

PIPAL

Source: Pipal consists of the dried fruits of *Piper longum* L. (Fam. Piperaceae),

Synonyms and Regional Names: Long Pepper· Ben. Pipul; Guj. Pipli; Hin. Piplamul, Pipal; Kan. Hippali; San. Pippali; Tam. Pippalu Tippili; Tel. Pipili.

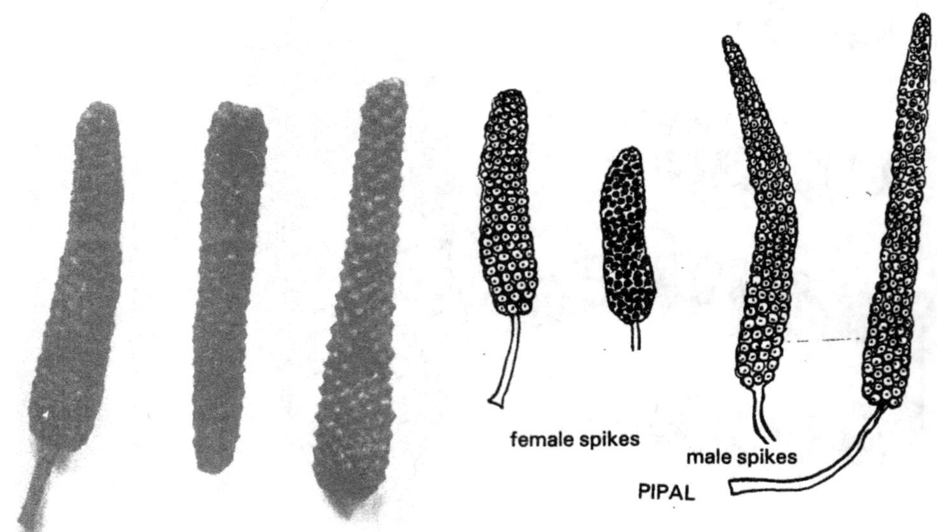

Morpholoyg: Form — very small, ovoid, completely sunk in solid fleshy spike; two types of spikes — male spike longer, slender 2.5 to 7.5 cm(l), female spikes short cylindrical 1.5 to 2.5 cm(l) and 5 to 7 mm(d); spikes are ovoid-oblong, erect, blunt, blackish green and shining; Odour — aromatic and Taste — pungent.

Active Constituents: ESSENTIAL OIL (1 to 2.5%) — responsible for the aroma — Terpenes like α and β-pinene, phellandrene, dipentene etc.

ALKALOIDS (5 to 9%) (acid amides) — responsible or pungency — piperine (1 – 2%), piperettine and chavicine, Some resins, starch etc.

Therapeutical and Pharmaceutical Uses: 1. Aromatic, stomachic and carminative 2. Alterative tonic (agent presumed to correct a disordered bodily function) 3. In acute and chronic bronchitis 4. Pipal is used in 135 drug preparations (Kapoor & Mitra).

PODOPHYLLUM

Source: Indian Podophyllum consists of the dried rhizomes and roots of *Podophyllum hexandrum* (Syn. *P. emodi* Wall) (Fam. Berberidaceae).

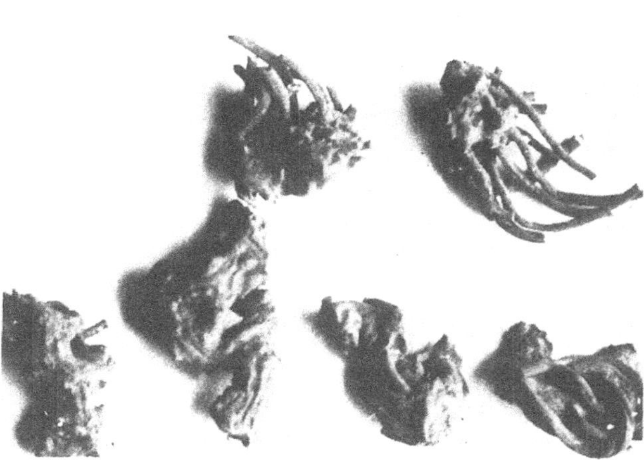

Synonyms and Regional Names

Guj. Veniwel

Hin. Popra, Papri,
 Bhavan bakra

Mar. Padwal

San. Laghupatha,
 Vakra

Morphology: Form – irregular, knotty, dorsiventrally flattened, contorted and tortuous pieces; Colour – yellowish brown to earthy brown; Size – 2 – 4 cm(l), 1 – 2 cm(t); Surface – on the upper side 3 – 4 cup shaped scars of aerial stems and leaves are seen, on the other side numerous stout roots are seen with longitudinal striations; Fracture – short and fractured surface – pale brown and starchy; Odour – slight and characteristic; Taste – bitter and acrid.

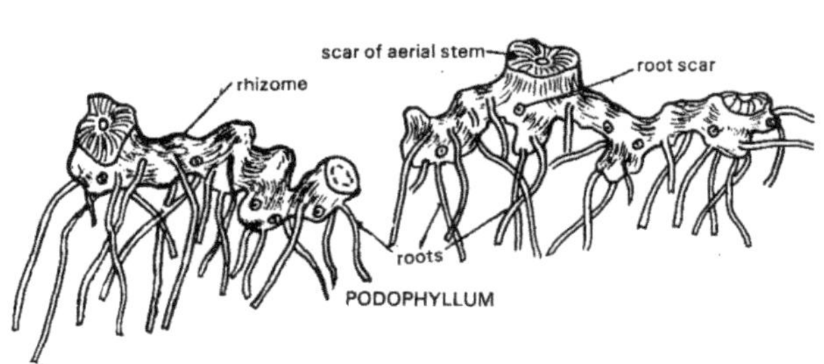

Active Constituents: RESINS (10 – 18%) – Lignan resin Podophyllin, a mixture containing – Podophyllotoxin (40%) – α-Peltatin – β-Peltatin in traces. FLAVONOID – Quercetin derivatives.

Therapeutical and Pharmaceutical Uses: 1. Highly toxic.   2. In the treatment of *Condylomata acuminatum* (soft, white warty outgrowth in the genital region).   3. Antimitotic effect – In cases of certain types of Cancer.   4. Violent cathartic (only the American variety but not the Indian Podophyllum).   5. A new synthetic derivative of podophyllotoxin – 'Etoposide' is used now to cure small cell – and testicular cancer.

Chemical Test

Macerate 0.5 g of powdered drug in 10 ml 90% alcohol for 10 min. and filter. A brown ppt. is obtained by adding 0.5 ml of conc. soln. of Copper acetate to the filtrate. American Podophyllum (*P. peltatum* Linn.) gives a green colour instead of brown ppt.

Adulterant: Puri and Jain (Planta Medica 1988, 269) report *Ainsliaea latifolia* (Fam. Asteraceae) as the adulterant of the Indian Podophyllum. The important differences are tabulated here.

Characters	Indian Podophyllum	Ainsliaea latifolia
Surface	wooly fibres absent	wooly fibres seen at the base of the stem
Fracture	starchy	horny
Taste	bitter and acrid	different
Vas. bundles	elongate radially	arranged in a ring
Trichomes	absent	arise from metaderm, simple fibre like with a swollen base
Resin cells	abundant	only a few cortical cells contain resin
Inulin	absent	present
Starch grains	abundant	rare
Crystals	present (?)	absent
Pith cells	not pitted	pitted
Add a few drops of strong soln. of copper acetate to the filtrate of the alcoholic extract	brown ppt.	greenish brown ppt.
Fluorescence	whole rhizome emits dark brown fluorescence	outer corky layer brown, the main body of the root and rhizome – white fluorescence.

PUDINA

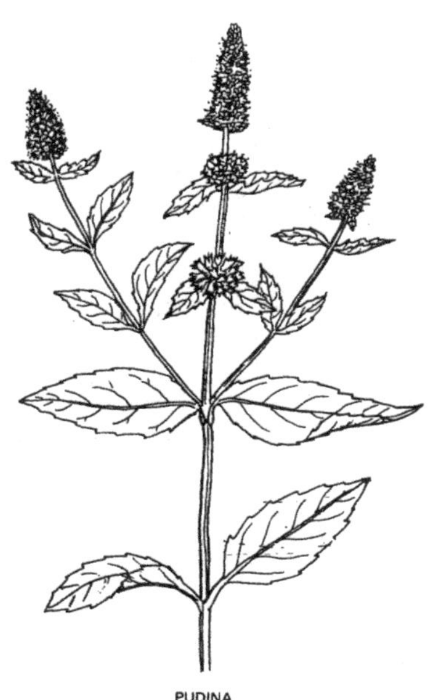

PUDINA

Source: Pudina consists of leaves and flowering tops of *Mentha spicata* Linn. Syn. *M. viridis* Linn. (Fam. Labiatae).

Synonyms and Regional Names: Spearmint, Japanese Mint, Mint, Ben. Guj. Kan. Mar. Tam. Tel. Pudina, Chutney maragu; Mal. Muthina.

Morphology: Pudina is glabrous perennial, 30 – 90 cm (h). Leaves sessile, lanceolate to ovate, acute, coarsely dentate, smooth on the upper side and glandular on the under side. Flowers are in spikes and lilac in colour. The leaves carry a characteristic aromatic odour and a mild pungent taste.

Active Constituents: VOLATILE OIL (0.2 to 0.5%) – l-carvone (50 – 60%), l-limonene, dipentene etc.

Nature of the Oil: Oil is colourless to yellow or greenish yellow liquid with characteristic aroma and spearment taste.

therapeutical and Pharmaceutical Uses: The herb is used as a stimulant, carminative and antispasmodic. Spearmint oil however is used for flavouring chewing gums, tooth pastes confectionary and pharmaceutical preparations.

PUNARNAVA

Source: Punarnava consists of the fresh or dried plant of *Boerhaavia diffusa* L. (Fam. Nyctaginaceae).

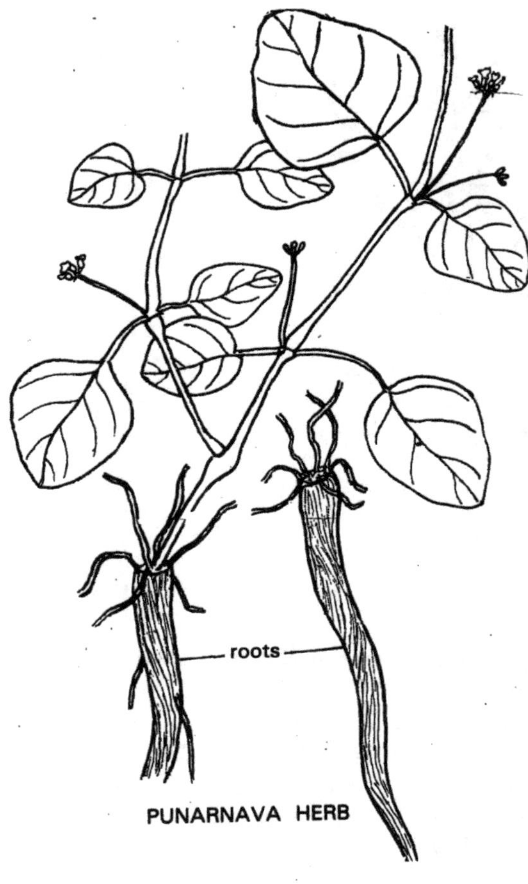

Synonyms and Regional Names: *B. repens,* Hog weed, Ben. Gandhpurna; Guj. Vakhakhaparo; Hin. Beshakapori; Kan. Sanadika, Komme, Gajjeru; Mal. Taludama, Tamilana; Mar. Punarnava; Tam. Chattarani, Mukkarattai; Tel. Galijeru, Attatamamidi.

Morphology: Perennial herb, pubescent or nearly glabrous with stout rootstock and many erect or procumbent branches. The tap root is long, fusiform and tapering. Stem prostrate or ascending, divaricately branched, slender, cylindrical, thickened at the nodes, often purplish. Leaves – at each node in unequal pairs, the larger 2.5 to 3.7 cm(l), the smaller 12 to 18 mm(l), both nearly as broad as long, ovate or sub-orbicular, rounded at apex, green and glabrous above but usually white with minute scales beneath. Margin entire somewhat undulate, often coloured pink, base rounded or subcordate, the slender petiole nearly as long as the blade, Flowers – small, pinkish red, 4 to 10 together in small umbels, arranged on slender long stalked corymbose, axillary or terminal panicles, bracteoles small, acute, perianth greenish on lower side, pinkish on the upper side, stamens 2 – 3, slightly exerted, Fruit – 6 mm(l), clavate, rounded broadly and bluntly 5 ribbed, viscidly glandular.

Active Constituents: ALKALOID (0.04%) – punarnavine, KNO_3, K_2SO_4, Chlorides etc. (6.5%).

STEROLS – β-sitosterol, α-sitosterol, palmitic acid, ester or β-sitosterol, tetracosanoic, hexacosanoic, stearic and archidic acids.

ALLANTOIN – a nitrogenous compound, Hentriacontane and ursolic acid.

Therapeutical and Pharmaceutical Uses: 1. Diuretic. 2. Extensively used in cases of edema and ascites (those due to early cirrhosis of liver and chronic peritonoitis). 3. Punarnava is used in 52 drug preparations (Kapoor & Mitra).

Punarnava is a controversial drug. Though *B. diffusa* is now well accepted all over as punarnava, *B. erecta, B. repens, B. repanda* and *B. verticillaster* are also used and sold as punarnava. To add to the confusion, *Trianthema decandra, T. pentandra, T. portulaceastrum* and *T. monogyna* (Fam. Ficoideae) also appear in market as punarnava.

PYRETHRUM

Source: Pyrethrum consists of the dried, closed or half open flower (flower heads) of *Chrysanthemum cinerariifolium* Vis. (Fam. Compositae). Pyrethrum contains not less than 0.7% of total pyrethrins (pyrethrin I and pyrethrin II).

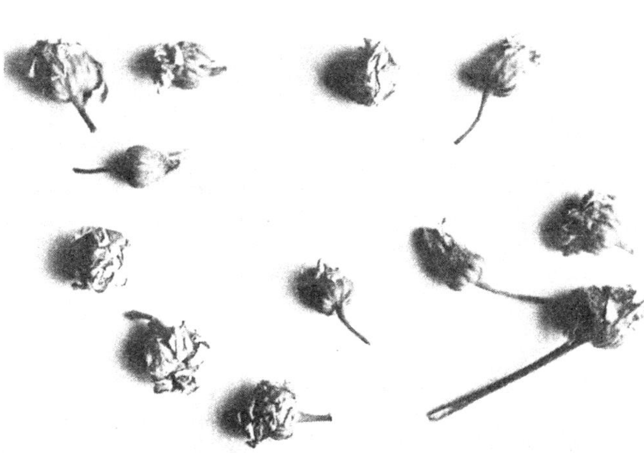

Synonym
Insect flower

Morphology
Type of inflorescence capitulum or head; Colour – yellow to yellowish brown; Size – 6 – 9 mm(d) when closed and 12 mm when open; Form – flower head hemi-spherical somewhat flat with 2 – 3 rows of involucral bracts which are lanceolate and thick.

Two types of florets are seen on the flower head; i) the ray (ligulate) florets forming the outer whorl. ii) Disc (tubular) florets occur in the centre. L. S. of Head; Receptacle – convex or nearly flat, devoid of paleae and measures 5 – 8 mm in

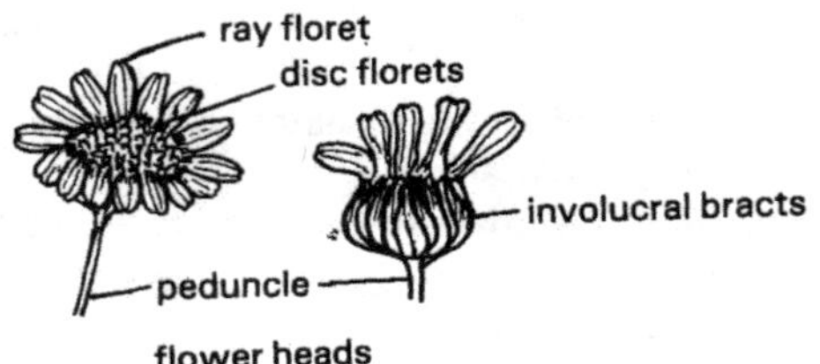

flower heads

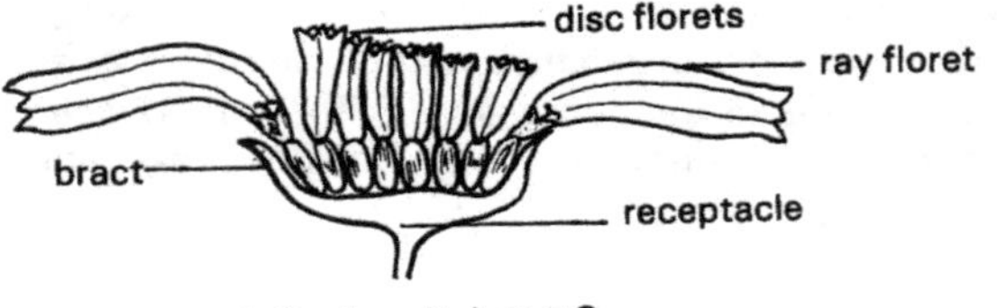

L.S. of capitulum × 3

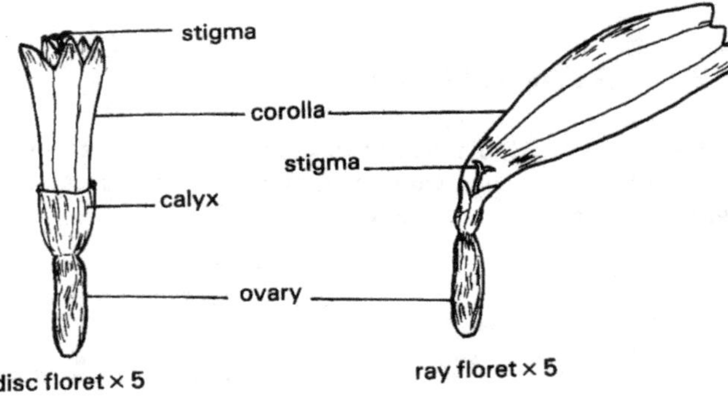

disc floret × 5   ray floret × 5

PYRETHRUM

diameter; Peduncle-short and longitudinally striated; Involucre – 3 rows of yellowish green bracts; outer bracts lanceolate, inner bracts spathulate, longer than the outer ones, bracts somewhat hairy on the outer surface. Ray florets-uniseriate 15 – 23, unisexual (pistillate); Corolla – cream or straw coloured, ligulate, oblong, gamopetalous, 3-small rounded teeth at the apex, the middle one being the smallest. Disc floret – 200 – 300, smaller in size, actinomorphic, bisexual and epigynous. Dalyx forms a thin whitish membranous tube. Corolla tubular, gamopetalous with 5 short tubes at the apex; Stamens-5, syngenesious (anthers united, filaments free), epipetalous, Gynoecium – oblong and inferior, style – short with bifid stigma: Odour – faint but characteristic and Taste – bitter,

Active Constituents

INSECTICIDES (0.4 – 2%) — Terpene esters
        — Pyrethrin I (0.64%) ⎫ Esters of
        — Pyrethrin II (0.65%) ⎬ Pyrethrolones
        — Cinerin I (0.15%) ⎫ Esters of
        — Cinerin II (0.23%) ⎬ Cinerolones
        — Jasmolin I ⎫ Esters of
        — Jasmolin II ⎬ Jasmolones

ESSENTIAL OIL (0.3%)

Therapeutical and Pharmaceutical Uses

1. Contact insecticide (Insects coming in contact with insecticides are killed) in the form of powder, sprays, aerosol, coil, cream and ointment.
2. To kill the human and animal skin parasites as well as intestinal parasites.
3. Used against flies and insect pests.

Substitutes and Adulterants: The reported adulterant is derived from the flower heads of *Chrysanthemum leucanthemum* (Ox-eye daisy). While the strap of the corolla of Pyrethrum flowers, have 17 veins and three rounded teeth of which the central one is smaller, that of the adulterant contains only 7 veins with 3 round teeth of which the centre one being the largest. Besides a calyx is absent in the adulterant.

QUASSIA

Source: Quassia is the dried stem wood of *Picrasma excelsa* (Sw.) Planch, *P. quassioides* Benth, *Picroena excelsa* (Sw. Lindly) or *P. quassioides* Benth or *Aeschrion excelsa* which is known in commerce as Jamaica quassia. (Fam. Simarubaceae).

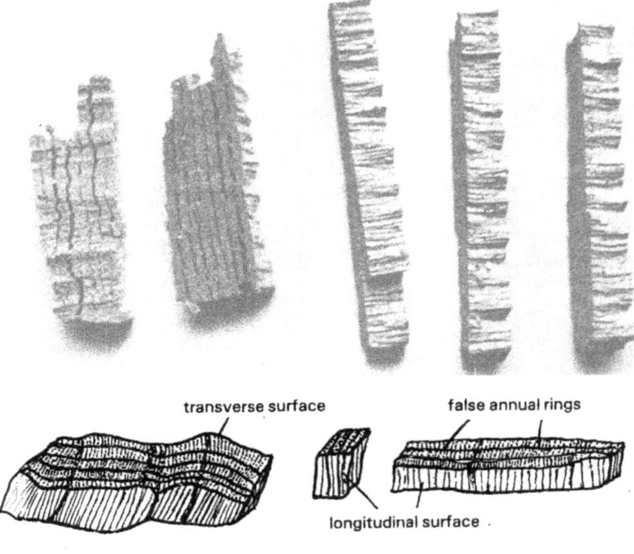

Synonyms and Regional Names
Quassia wood, Jamaica quassia; Hin. Bharangi; San. Charangi

Morphology
Condition – dry and Size – variable;
Form – chips, raspings or shavings, light, tough bit splits easily;
Colour – yellowish or yellowish white;
Surface – appearance of false annual rings;
No odour but intensely bitter in taste.

Active Constituents: BITTER PRINCIPLES OF TERPENOID NATURE
– Quassin – Picrasmin or Isoquassin – Neoquassin

Therapeutical and Pharmaceutical Uses: 1. Bitter tonic 2. To expel thread worms 3. Insecticide (against flies) 4. Tincture quassia is used against ouse 5. To denature alcohol.

Substitutes and Adulterants: Surinam quassia (*Quassia amara*) official in Continent is used as a substitute as it contains the bitter principles – quassin and neoquassin. It is possible to differentiate one from the other by microscopic means. While the meduallary ray cells in Jamaican quassia are 2 – 3 cells wide, in Surinam quassia about 60% of the ray cells are one cell wide. Further, calcium oxalate crystals are absent in Surinam quassia but present in the wood parenchyma of Jamaican species. Exhausted quassia from which the bitter principles have been removed, is used as an adulterant. The exhausted sample will have low aqueous extract (2.7%) while that of the genuine sample would vary from 6.3 to 8.6%.

QUILLAIA

Source: Quillaia is the dried inner bark of *Quillaia saponaria* Molina and of other species of *Quillaia* (Fam. Rosaceae).

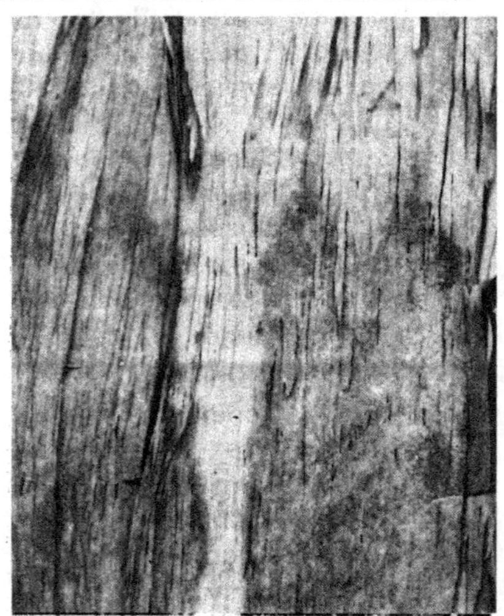

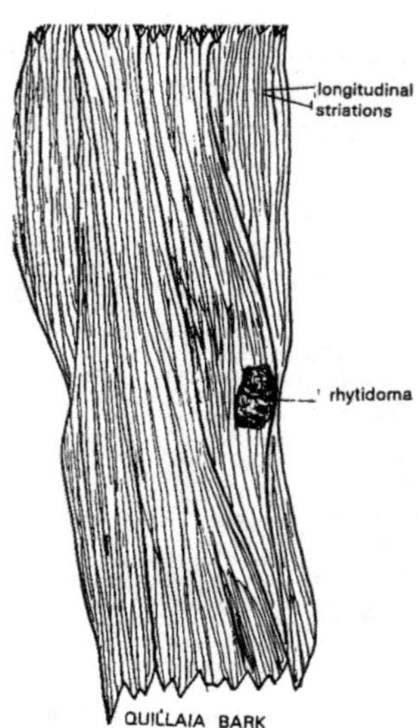

Synonyms: Soap bark, Panama wood.

Morphology: Condition – dry; Shape – flat strips; Size – varies upto 1 m(l), 20 cm(b) and 3 – 10 mm(t); Colour – outer surface brownish white with reddish white patches of rhytidoma and inner surface yellowish white. Outer surface also shows longitudinal striations; Fracture – laminated and splintery; Odour – none but the powdered drug is sternutatory; Taste – acrid and astringent.

Active Constituents

SAPONINS – Tritepenoid saponins (10%)
      – Quillaic acid (genin or aglycone)
      – Galacturonic acid ⎤
      – Glucuronic acid ⎬ sugars
      – Galactose   ⎦

Therapeutical and Pharmaceutical Uses: 1. In the soap industry as-detergents, shampoo etc. 2. Emulsifying agent (in the preparation of coal tar emulsions). 3. In tooth paste and powder.

RASNA

Source: Rasna consists of the rhizomes of *Alpinia officinarum* Hance (Fam. Zingiberaceae) obtained from 4 to 10 years old plants, washed, trimmed, cut into segments and carefully dried. It consists of not less than 0.5% of volatile oil.

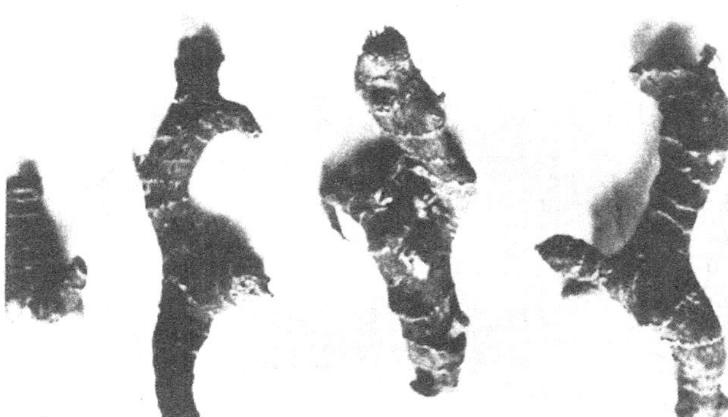

Synonyms and Regional Names

Ben. Sugandha
    bacha
Hin. Khulinjan
Kan. Rasagadde
Mal. Aratta
Tam. Chitrattai
Tel. Sannaraashtramu

Morphology: Form — cylindrical, irregularly branched and often bent like knee; Size — 5 – 10(l), and upto 2 cm(t); Colour — copper red externally, Cinnamon brown internally; Surface — marked with fine annuli of lighter colour than the general surface; Odour — aromatic; Taste — characteristic spicy, aromatic and pungent; Fracture — fibrous and tough.

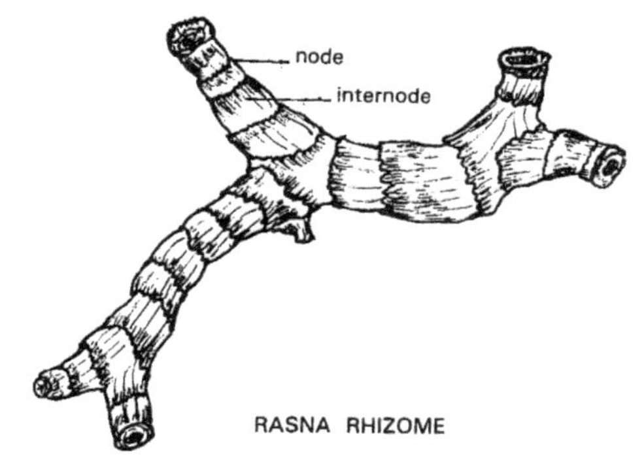

RASNA RHIZOME

Active Constituents

ESSENTIAL OIL (0.5 – 1%)	– cineole, α-pinene, eugenol
	– sesquiterpenes – sesquiterpene alcohol
RESIN	– Alpinol or galangol
TANNINS	– Phlobaphenes
FLAVONOIDS	– Kaempferide, galangin and alpinin

Therapeutical and Pharmaceutical Uses: 1. Stomachic, stimulant and carminative
2. In rheumatism and catarrhal affections, specially in bronchial catarrh.
3. Antibacterial and antifungal (flavonoids) + Essential oil.
(Planta Medica 1981,2, 140).

RAUWOLFIA

Rauwolfia consists of the dried roots of *Rauwolfia serpentina* Benth ex. Kurz (Fam. Apocynaceae) with the bark intact, collected in autumn from three to four years old plants. It contains not less than 0.15% of reserpine group of alkaloids, calculated as reserpine.

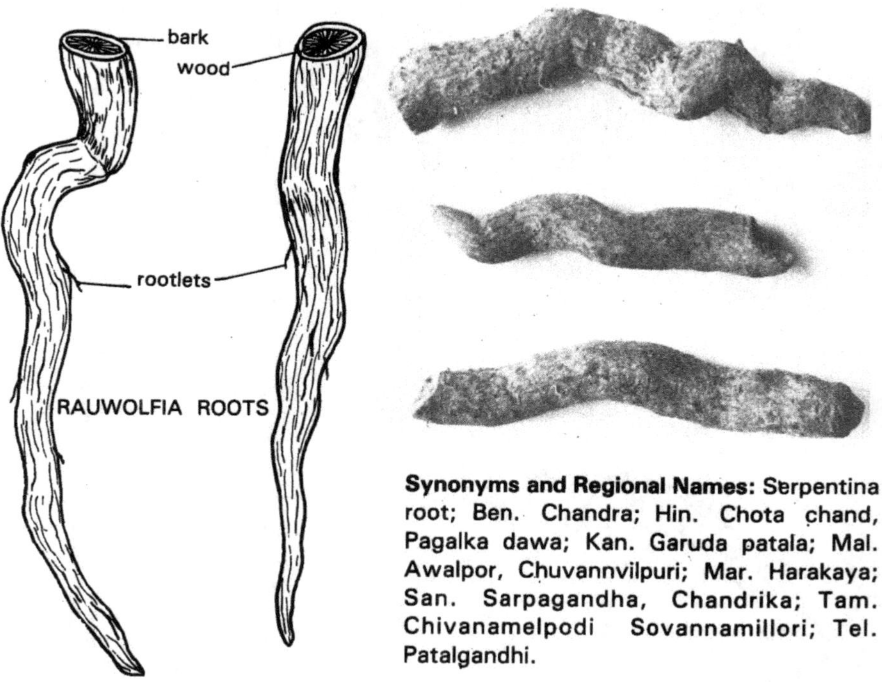

Synonyms and Regional Names: Serpentina root; Ben. Chandra; Hin. Chota chand, Pagalka dawa; Kan. Garuda patala; Mal. Awalpor, Chuvannvilpuri; Mar. Harakaya; San. Sarpagandha, Chandrika; Tam. Chivanamelpodi Sovannamillori; Tel. Patalgandhi.

Morphology: External features of roots and rhizomes are nearly similar but rhizomes can be made out by the presence of small central pith. Drug consists of mostly small pieces which are 2 – 15 cm long and 3 to 22 mm diameter. Pieces are cylindrical, slightly tapering and tortuous. Outer surface is greyish yellow, pale brown or brown. Fracture short and fractured surface shows yellowish to brown bark and dense pale yellow radiating wood with 2 to 8 annular rings occupying nearly three fourth of the diameter. Rauwolfia has no odour but bitter taste.

Microscopy (Transverse Section)

T. S. of the root presents a circular outline with typical stratified cork and other secondary features. Following are the tissues seen from the periphery to the centre.

PERIDERM

Cork (Phellem) stratified, consists of alternating bands – of smaller, suberized and un-lignified cells upto 8 – 10 rows in radial depth and – of larger, suberized but lignified cells upto 5 – 7 rows in radial depth.

Phellogen indistinct but is seen as a narrow layer of thin walled cells.

Phelloderm 5 – 7 layers, immediately below the phellem, cells are arranged in radial rows whereas away from phellem, cells are oval and have intercellular spaces. Phelloderm contains abundant starch grains (with triradiate hilum) and typical twin prisms of calcium oxalate.

SECONDARY PHLOEM is traversed by conspicuous medullary rays. Phloem consists of sieve tubes, companion cells and phloem parenchyma. Starch grains and calcium oxalate prisms (as twins and in groups) occur throughout the phloem tissue.

SECONDARY XYLEM is also traversed by well developed medullary rays. Xylem consists of vessels, wood fibres and lignified parenchyma. The vessels appear rounded, polygonal or at times radially elongated and occur either single or in pairs. Xylem fibres appear as rounded or polygonal structures with thick lignified walls. Typical oxalate prisms and starch grains resembling those of the phelloderm and phloem occur freely in the wood parenchyma.

MEDULLARY RAYS run radially from the centre to the cortex through the phloem. Rays in the xylem region are lignified, pitted and are 1 – 5 cells wide although uniseriate rays are prominent. In the phloem region the ray cells are not lignified. Starch and typical oxalate prisms are present in the medullary ray cells.

Active Constituents

ALKALOIDS – Indole alkaloids (1.5 or 3%) present mostly in bark.

Weakly basic Indole type (pH 7 to 7.5)

– **Reserpine** group – Reserpine – Rescinnamine – Deserpidine

Tertiary Indoline Alkaloids (pH 8)

– **Ajmaline** group – Ajmaline – Ajmalicine

Strongly Basic Anhydronium Bases (pH 11)

Serpentine group – Serpentine – Serpentinine – Alstonine

Therapeutical and Pharmaceutical Uses: 1. Sedative – calms down activities and excitement (Reserpine **Group**) 2. Stimulates the central of peripheral nervous systems (Ajmaline **Group**). 3. Antihypertensive (decreases blood pressure) (Serpentine **Group**).

Substitutes and Adulterants: The following species of *Rauwolfia* are substituted for the genuine drug. 1. *R. vomitoria.* This can be distinguished from the offical drug on the basis of sclereids which are present here in abundance. 2. *R. canescens.*

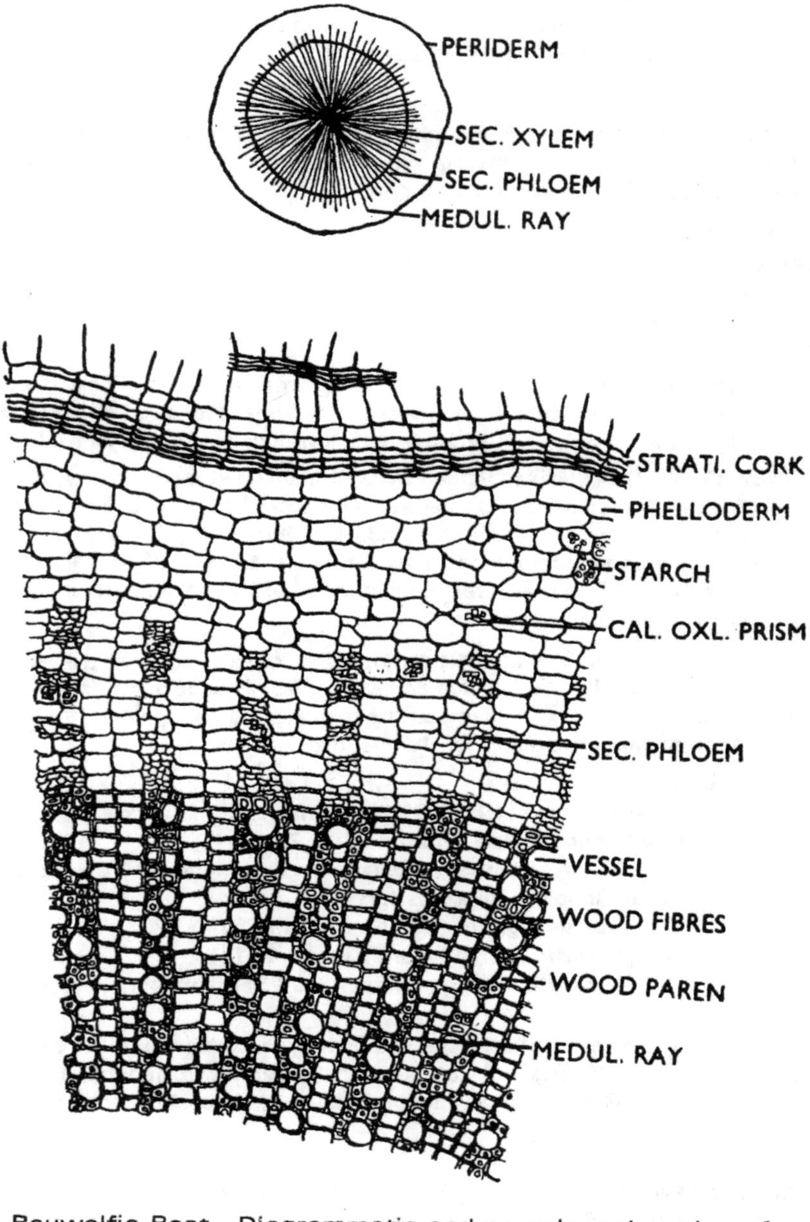

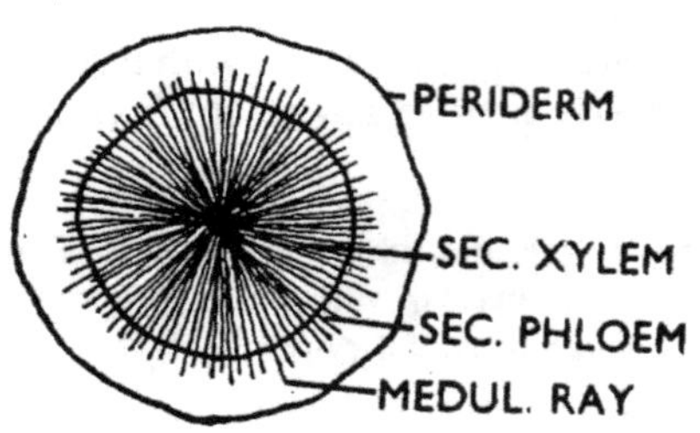

Rauwolfia Root. Diagrammatic and an enlarged portion of
T. S. (X 100)

Here again the stone cells are present but the characteristic stratified cork is totally absent. 3. *R. micrantha* shows both stratified cork and stone cells. All these do contain reserpine and other less important alkaloids in small quantities. Roots and rhizomes of two other species namely – *R. densiflora* and *R. perakensis* do not contain reserpine and therefore to be considered as adulterants. They do have stratified cork and stone·cells.

RHUBARB

Source: Indian Rhubarb consists of the dried rhizome of *Rheum emodi* Wall and *R. webbianum* (Fam. Polygonaceae). It is collected usually from 6 to 7 years old plants just before the flowering season and marketed with cortex intact or partially decorticated. Chinese Rhubarb is obtained from *R. palmatum* and *R. officinale.*

Synonyms and Regional Names: Rhizoma Rhei; Ben. Resu-chini; Guj. Gamni revanchini; Hin. Revandchine; Kan. Revakinni; Mal. Variyatta; San. Banglachini, Gandhini Pita; Tam. Mattirevalchini; Tel. Nattu-revalchinni.

Morphology: Shape – compact solid, somewhat cylindrical, barrel shaped, conical or plano-convex pieces; Size – variable, 2 – 20 cm(l), 1.5 – 8 cm(d); Colour – orange brown; Surface – irregularly longitudinally wrinkled, furrowed or ridged with a brownish or yellowish brown cortex; Fracture – granular and uneven; Fractured surface – starch present; transverse surface usually shows a prominent cambium line, annulations, 'star spots' (abnormal vascular bundles) the latter though

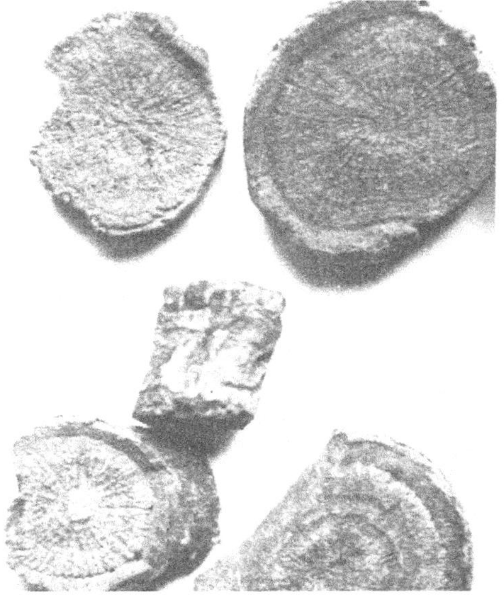

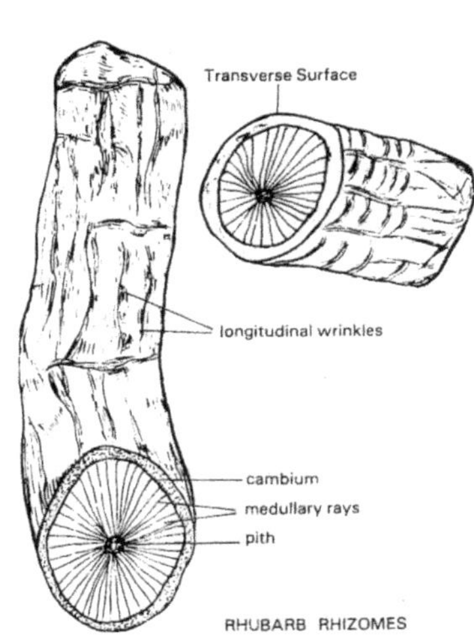

not in Indian species; and at times drying holes. Fine yellow powder often covers the transverse surface; Odour – characteristic; Taste – bitter and slightly astringent.

Active Constituents: GLYCOSIDES – Anthracene derivatives – (2 – 3%), 8 – O – mono and diglycosides of chrysophanol, aloe-emodin, rhein, emodin and physcion; Heterodianthrones like palmidin A, B, C and rheidin A, B, C etc. TANNINS – Glucogallin – Tetrarin, Catechin and Epicatechin. RESINS, FATTY OIL etc.

Therapeutical and Pharmaceutical Uses: 1. Laxative 2. In small doses as antidiarrhoetic.

Chemical Test: Constituents answer Borntrager's test. For details see Senna.

Substitutes and Adulterants: Officially there is no particular mention of an adulterant or a substitute. However, the following may be considered as substitutes as they contain the anthracene derivatives.

1. Chinese Rhapontic Rhubarb (*Rheum rhaponticum*) 2. English Rhubarb (*Rheum officinale*).

SATAVARI

Source: Satavari consists of the tuberous roots of *Asparagus racemosus* Willd. (Fam. Liliaceae).

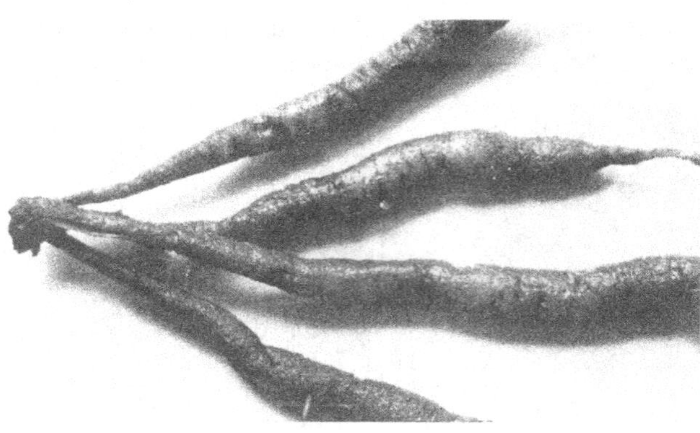

Synonyms and Regional Names
Ben. Satmuli
Guj. Satavar
Hin. Shakakul
    satavari
Kan. Shatavari
Mal. Shatavali
Mar. Shatavarimull
Tam. Tannirvittan-
    kizhangu
Tel. Philli-gaga,
    Tsallogadda

Morphology: Type – fasiculated; Form – adventitious roots arising from a single point, become fleshy and tuberous, tapering towards the base and swollen at the middle; Colour – silver white or light ash in colour; Size – 5 – 15 cm(!) and maximum diameter 1 – 2 cm; Surface – more or less smooth in fresh samples and fine longitudinal wrinkles in dry samples; Fracture – complete.

Active Constituents: GLYCOSIDES
— Saponin glycosides – Saponin A_4, A_5, A_6, A_7, A_8
— Saponin A_4 yields on hydrolysis sarasapogenin, glucose and rhamnose.

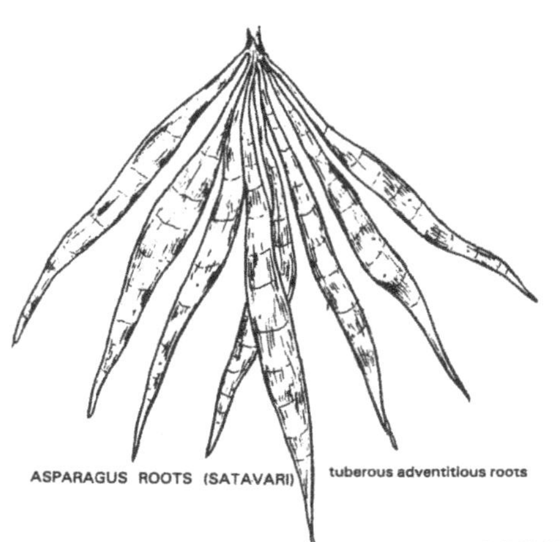

SAUSSUREA

Source: Saussurea consists of the dried roots of *Saussurea lappa* Clarke (Fam. Compositae).

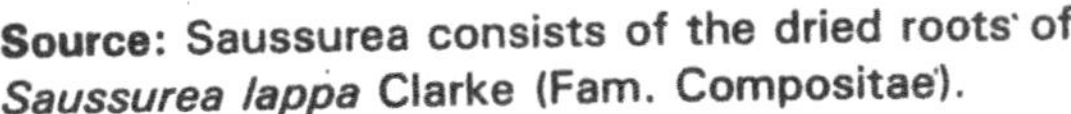

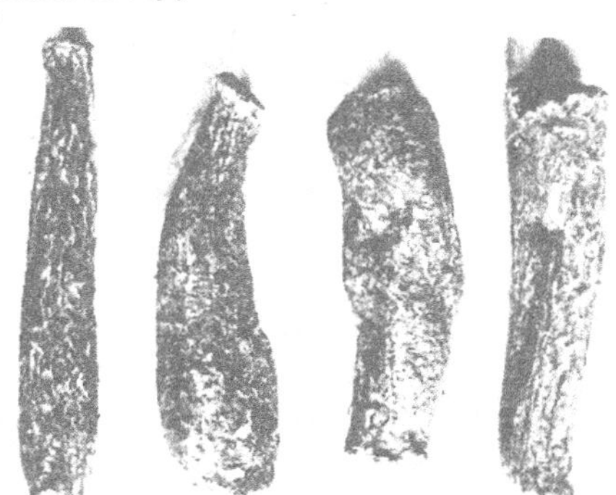

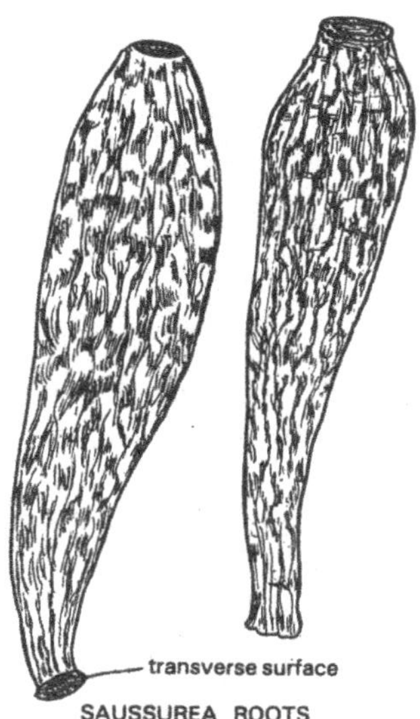

Synonyms and Regional Names: Costus, Ben. Kur; Guj. Kut; Hin. Pachak; Mal. Sappudi; San. Agada kushtha; Tam. Tel. Koshtam

Morphology: Form – thick, light, straight and stout; Colour – dull, rusty red or blackish brown; Size – 2.4 to 7.5 cm(l), 2.5 to 3.7 cm(b); Surface – tubercle like short protruberances on the outer surface. Cut surface shows (a) the outer thin region containing epiblema and pericycle (b) the middle woody portion of a lighter colour showing fine radial striations and (c) inner central region. Fracture – short; horny; Odour – strong, aromatic and characteristic; Taste – somewhat bitter.

Active Constituents: VOLATILE OIL (1.5 to 2.5%) – Costunolide a new sesquiterpene lactone – methoxy dihydro constunolide.
RESINOIDS, ALKALOIDS and TANNINS.

Therapeutical and Pharmaceutical Uses: 1. Stimulant in cough, asthma, fever, dyspepsia and skin diseases.   2. In high class perfumery.

SENEGA

Source: Indian Senega consists of the roots of *Polygala chinensis*. Linn. collected in autumn from 3 – 4 year old plants (Fam. Polygalaceae).

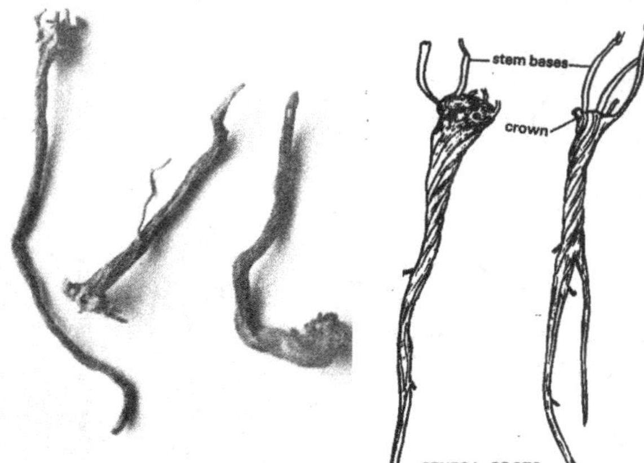

Synonyms and Regional Names
Chinensis root
Guj. Pilibhonya sana
Hin. Meradu
Mar. Negli

Morphology
Shape – long, tapering with knotty crown bearing numerous buds and bases of aerial stems;

Size – 5 – 20 cm(l), 2 – 10 mm(d); Colour – light brown; Surface – marked with longitudinal striations; Fracture – short; Odour – characteristic; Taste – bitter and acrid.

Active Constituents: SAPONIN – Triterpenoid saponin – Polygallic acid (4.5%) – Senegin (4%) yielding on hydrolysis Presenegenin and galactose, rhamnose, xylose and fucose as sugars.

Therapeutical and Pharmaceutical Use: Expectorant (removes the catarrhal matter and phlegm from bronchial tubes) in case of bronchitis.

Substitutes and Adulterants: The official Senega is derived from *P. senega* indigenous to USA but now cultivated in Japan. The roots of *Andrachne aspera* (Euphorbiaceae) is said to be according to some as Pakistan Senega. *Glinus oppositifolia* (Aizoaceae) also sold as Indian Senega does contain saponins and starch as well. The vascular bundles however appear in concentric rings.

Note: Thus there is certainly some confusion about the authenticity of Indian Senega and as such no final word can be said here.

SENNA

Source: Indian Senna consists of the dried leaflets and fruits of *Cassia angustifolia* Vahl. known in commerce as Tinnevelly senna (Fam. Leguminosae).

Synonyms and Regional Names: Indian Senna, Tinnevelly senna; Ben. Sonamukhi; Guj. Nat-ki-sana; Hin. Sunnamaki, Sana-ka-pat; Nelavarike; Mal. Nila Vaka; Mar. Sonamukhi; San. Swarnamuki, Bhumiari; Tam. Nilavarai; Tel. Sunamukhi.

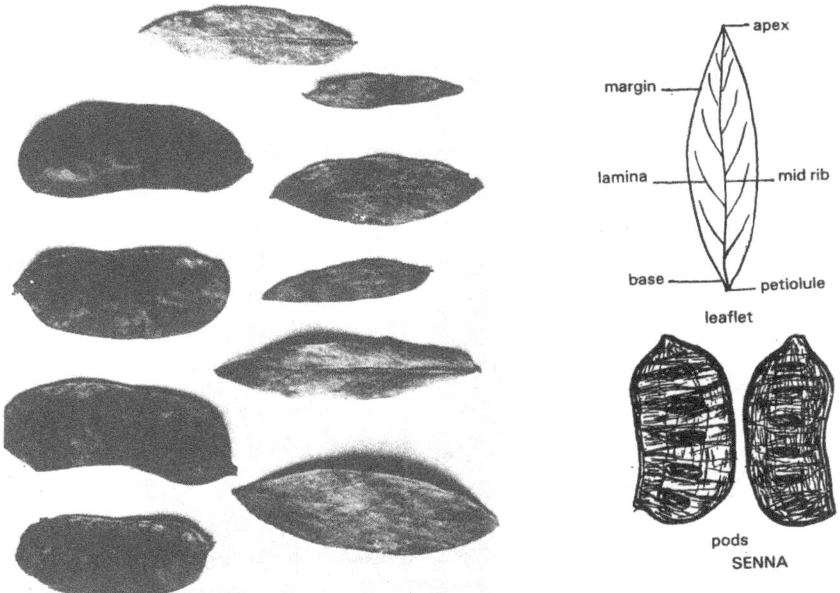

Morphology: Condition – dry; Type – a leaflet of paripinnately compound leaf; Shape – lanceolate or ovate laneolate; Size – 2.5 – 6 cm(l) and 7 – 8 mm (w); Petiole – a small petiolule present; Margin entire; Apex – mucronate; Base slightly asymmetrical; Venation – pinnately reticulate; Up. Surface – pale green or yellowish green and glabrous; Low. Surface-shows prominent transverse lines; Odour – none; Taste – mucilaginous and slightly bitter.

Fruit: Type – legume; Shape – broadly oblong, flat, thin or somewhat reniform with more rounded apex, exhibiting the remains of style; Colour – brownish green; Size – about 5 cm(l) and 2 cm(b); Odour – slight; Taste – somewhat bitter.

Microscopy (Transverse Section)

T. S. of a leaflet shows an isobilateral condition. The following are the tissues represented in the lamina and the midrib region:

LAMINA

Upper epidermis Single layered with polygonal cells covered on the outside by a thick warty cuticle. Some epidermal cells contain mucilage. Only covering trichomes emerge from the epidermal layer. Trichomes are non-glandular short, thick,

111

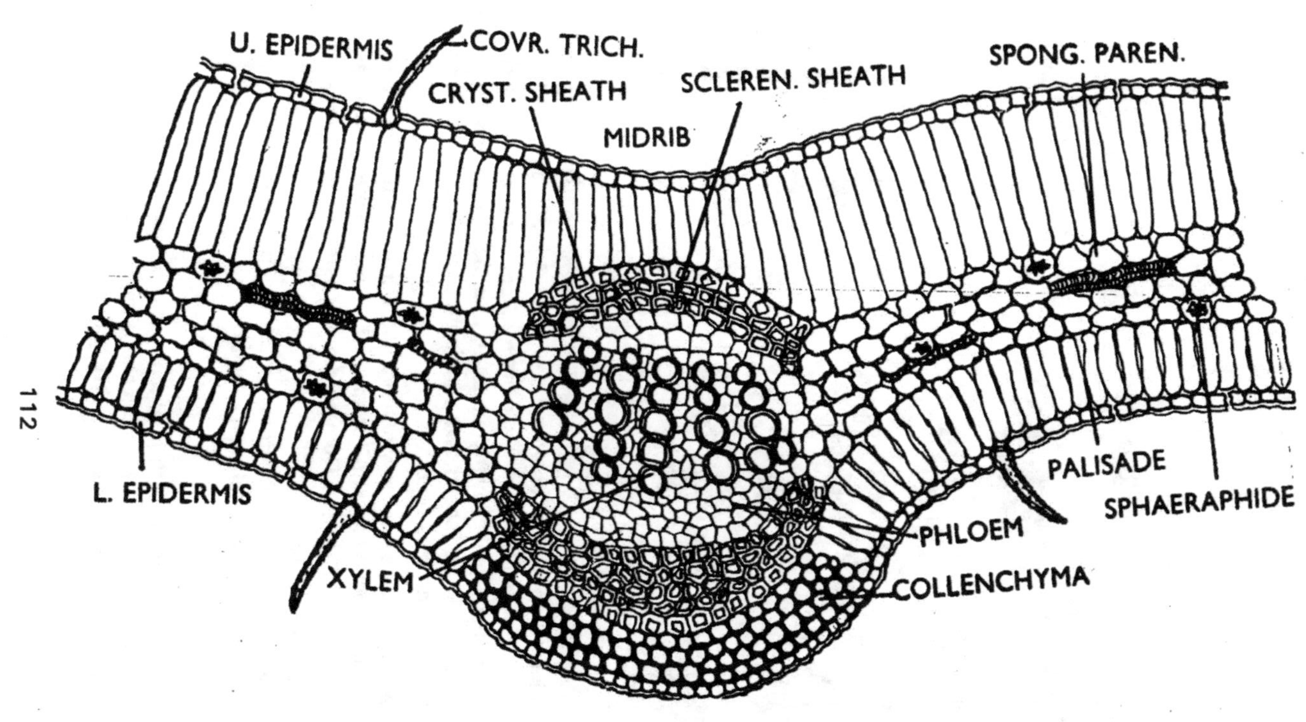

Senna Leaflet T. S. (×100)

unicellular, nonlignified, warty and slightly curved at the bulbous base. Stomata are seen at regular intervals.

Mesophyll is differentiated into palisade and spongy parenchyma. Being a unifacial or isobilateral leaf, palisade is further differentiated into upper and lower palisade.

Upper palisade single layered, compact with elongated, narrow, columnar cells and this continues also over the midrib region.

Spongy parenchyma thin, narrow, loosely arranged between the upper and lower palisade. Vascular strands are seen very frequently. Few sphaeraphides are also seen in the parenchyma.

Lower palisade is restricted, unlike upper palisade, to lamina region only. Cells are smaller than those of upper palisade, loosely arranged and their walls are wavy.

Lower epidermis is very similar to upper epidermis.

MIDRIB presents a flat ventral surface and convex dorsal surface. The epidermal layers are continuous over the midrib. The cells of the lower epidermis however are small with thick cuticle. The cells of the upper palisade, a tissue which appears below the upper epidermis in the midrib region, are relatively smaller. As mentioned earlier the lower palisade is not represented in the midrib and instead a patch of collenchyma is seen.

Collateral vascular bundle is prominent occupying the central portion of the midrib. Xyelm as usual is towards the ventral surface and pholem towards the dorsal surface. The vascular bundle is covered on both the sides (dorsal and ventral) by patches of sclerenchymatous fibres. Characteristic of Folia Senna is that these fibres are ensheathed by a layer of parenchyma, the individual cells of which contain calcium oxalate prisms. Such fibres with crystal sheath can also be seen, if not frequently, in the lamina region.

Surface preparation shows typical characteristic Rubiaceous stomata and polygonal epidermal cells and covering trichomes.

Active Constituents

GLYCOSIDES — Anthracene glycosides ⎤
               — Dianthrone glycosides ⎦ Leaves 3% (Pods 1.5 to 2.5%)
               — Sennoside A (0.3 to 0.45%) ⎤ Homodianthrone
               — Sennoside B (0.3 to 0.5%) ⎦ glycosides
               — Sennoside C and ⎤
                  Sennoside D ⎦ Heterodianthrone glycosides
      — Rhein, Aloe emodin — aglycones
FLAVONOID — Kaempferol glycoside

Anthraquinone Test or Borntrager's Test: Boil about 100 mg of powdered drug in 5 ml 10% H_2SO_4 for one or two minutes. As a result O-glycosides present undergo hydrolysis. Filter immediately. The cooled filtrate is now extracted in a separating funnel with organic solvent like ether, chloroform or benzene. The organic solvent layer is separated by a pipette and to this 5 ml of 10% ammonia is added. Shake gently and then allow to separate. The formation of a rose-pink coloration in the upper ammoniacal layer indicates the presence of anthraquinones.

Therapeutical and Pharmaceutical Use: Laxative, used specially in case of habitual constipation.

Substitutes and Adulterants: Wild plants of *Cassia angustifolia* growing in Arabia also called Mecca, Bombay and Arabian Senna are considered, as a substitute as they are therapeutically active. The leaflets are narrower and elongated and resemble, to a certain extent that of Indian Senna. It is reported that on the basis of vein-islet number, this species can be differentiated from other species. One another species to be considered as a substitute as it contains the active principles the anthraquinone derivatives is *C. obovata*. As per the species name the leaflets are obovate and distinct from the official drug. Leaflets of *C. auriculata* (Palthe Senna) is an adulterant of Indian Senna. The trichomes of these are three times longer. It does not contain any anthraquinones as in official drug but contains leuco-anthocyanidin which is responsible for two specific colour reactions. When boiled with chloral hydrate crimson colour is obtained and with 80% H_2SO_4 red colour.

SESAME OIL

Source: Sesame Oil is the fixed oil obtained by expression from the seeds of *Sesamum indicum* L. (Fam. Pedaliaceae).

Synonyms and Regional Names: Gingelly oil, Ben. Tiler tel; Guj. Mithu tel; Hin. Til ka tel; Kan. Ellu-enne; San. Tila taila; Tam. Nallennai; Tel. Manchi nune.

Nature: Colour – pale yellow; Consistency – oily liquid; Odour – somewhat pleasant; Taste – bland.

Active Constituents: LIPIDS (45-60%)
– Fixed Oil – mixture of glycerides – the fatty acid constituents of which are oleic and linoleic acids and a small percentage of palmitic, stearic acid etc.
– Sesamolin, a lignan of the unsaponifiable portion of the oil. Sisamolin on hydrolysis yields sesamol a phenolic constituent responsible for the excellent stability of the oil.

Therapeutical and Pharmaceutical Uses: 1. Pharmaceutical aid.   2. As a solvent for intramuscular injections.   3. Nutritive, laxative, demulcent and emollient. 4. An effective synergist for pyrethrum insecticides.

Chemical Test: On shaking 1 ml of sesame oil with a soln. of 0.5 g of sucrose in 10 ml HCl for half a min. the acid layer becomes bright red changing to dark red on standing (distinction from most of the other fixed oils).

SHANKHPUSHPI

Source: Shankhpushpi consists of the dried plant of *Evolvulus alsinoides* L. (Fam. Convolvulaceae).

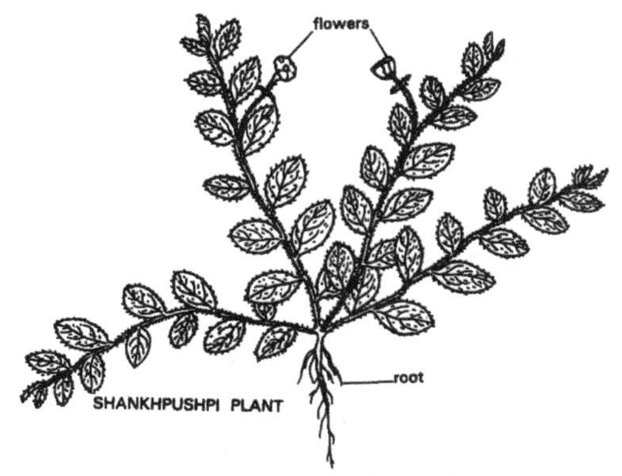

Synonyms and Regional Names

Hin.	Shankhpushpi
Kan.	
Mal.	Vishnukranti
San.	
Tel.	
Mar.	Shankhvalli
Tam.	Vishnukrandi

Morphology: A hairy perennial herb, prostrate wiry branches arising from a small woody root-stock, leaves simple, nearly sissile, alternate, lanceolate, oblong – ovate or even suborbicular; Flowers – light blue, mostly solitary; Fruit – four angled capsule.

Active Constituents: ALKALOIDS – Betaine, evolvine and one another water soluble base. The water extract also contains proteins, aminoacids, carbohydrates, phenolic compounds, sugars and tannins.

Therapeutical and . Pharmaceutical Uses: 1. Bitter tonic. 2. In dysentery. 3. Leaves made into cigarettes and smoked in chronic bronchitis and asthma. 4. Anthelmintic and antiphlogistic (diminishing inflammation). 5. Sedative.

Note: Four more plants are also named as Shankhpushpi and these are (1) *Clitoria ternatea* (2) *Canscora decussata* and (3) *Crotalaria verrucosa* (4) *Convolvulus pluricaulis, C. microphyllus*. In other words, 'shankhpuspi' is a highly controversial drug and as such its correct identity to this date is not known and *E. alsinoides* is only one possibility.

SHARK-LIVER OIL

Source: Shark-liver Oil is the oil obtained from the fresh or carefully preserved livers of the shark—*Hypoprion brevirostris*. It contains in 1 g not less than 6000 International Units of Vitamin 'A' activity.

Nature: Colour – pale yellow to brownish yellow; Odour – fishy and Taste – fishy and bland; Solubility – miscible in light petroleum (50° – 60°), ether, chloroform and slightly soluble in alcohol.

Active Constituents: Vitamin A and glycerides of saturated and unsaturated fatty acids. The concentration of Vitamin A ranges from 15000 to 30000 units per gram.

Therapeutical and Pharmaceutical Uses: 1. Source of Vitamin A. 2. In the treatment of Xerophthalmia (abnormal dryness of the surface of the conjuctiva). 3. In combination with Vitamin D, it is given as a tonic and nutritive in cases of TB.

Chemical Tests: Owing to the presence of Vitamin A the following tests are performed: 1) drop of shark-liver oil is dissolved in 1 ml of chloroform. Addition of 1 or 2 drops of H_2SO_4 and shaking thereafter results in a pale violet colour which finally changes to brown or blue colour. 2) 1 ml of the shark-liver oil is dissolved in 10 ml of chloroform and thereafter treated with a saturated soln. of antimony trichloride in chloroform. On shaking a blue colour is formed.

STARCH

Source: Starch consists of polysaccharide granules obtained from the grains of maize *Zea mays* L. or of rice *Oryza sativa* L. or of wheat *Triticum aestivum* L. (Fam. Graminae) or from the tubers of the potato — *Solanum tuberosum* L. (Fam. Solanaceae).

Chemical Constituents: CARBOHYDRATES — Polysaccharides
— Water soluble 'Amylose'   — Water insoluble 'Amylopectin'
'Amylose and Amylopectin' are two structurally different polysaccharides.

Amylose is a linear molecule consisting of 250-300 glucose units. Amylopectin consists of 300-1000 or more glucose units. Amylopectin is both linear and branched at points. Pasty nature and adhesive property of starch is due to Amylopectin.

Therapeutical and Pharmaceutical Uses: 1. It is mainly used as a dusting power 2. As a pharmaceutical aid. 3. Used as an antidote for iodine poisoning. 4. Source of food-nutrition. 5. Protective and demulcent. 6. In paper-sizing and textile industry and in laundry practice etc. 7. It is the starting product from which liquid glucose, dextrose, dextrins are made. 8. Acts as a basis for identification of drugs in Pharmacognosy.

Chemical Test: Boil a few mg of starch powder in 10 ml of water. On cooling a translucent viscous fluid or jelly is observed which turns deep blue on addition of solution of iodine. The colour disappears on warming and re-appears on cooling.

STORAX

Source: Storax is the purified balsam obtained from the wounded stem of *Liquidambar orientalis* Miller (Fam. Hamamelidaceae).

Synonyms and Regional Names: Purified or prepared Storax, Levant Storax, Liquid Storax, Ben. Guj. Hin. Kan. Mar. Shilaras, Mal. Rasamalla, San. Silhaka, Tam. Neri-arishippal, Tel. Shilaras.

Nature: Form — viscous liquid; Colour — transparent; Odour and Taste — balsamic and agreeable; Solubility — insoluble in water while soluble in alcohol and ether.

Active Constituents: RESIN COMBINATIONS/BALSAMIC ACIDS (BALSAM)
– Cinnamic acid (16 – 24%) – Cinnamic acid ester – Storesinol (25%)

Therapeutical and Pharmaceutical Use: Pharmaceutical aid (Antiseptic).

Chemical Tests: 1. On warming 0.5 g of the drug in 1 ml of chloral hydrate, a clear soln. is obtained.- 2. On warming a well shaken mixture of 1 g storax + 2 ml potassium chromate + 1 ml H_2SO_4 an odour of benzaldehyde is produced. 3. On warming a mixture of 1 g storax + 4 ml of 2% $KMnO_4$, a benzaldehyde odour is produced.

STROPHANTHUS

Source: Strophanthus consists of dried ripe seeds of *Strophanthus kombe* (Oliv) freed from the awns and as well from *S. gratus* (Wall. et Hook). (Fam. Apocynaceae).

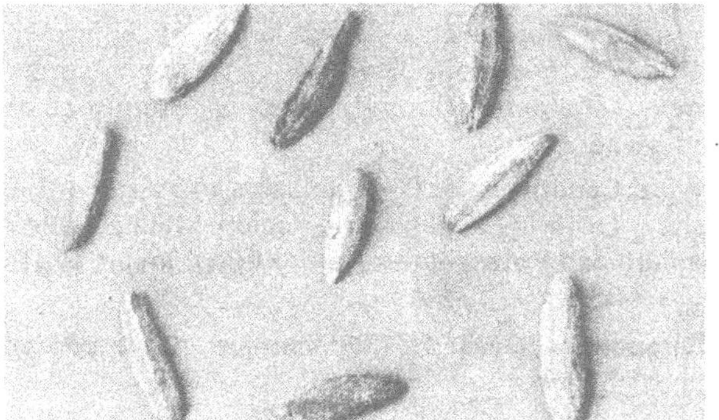

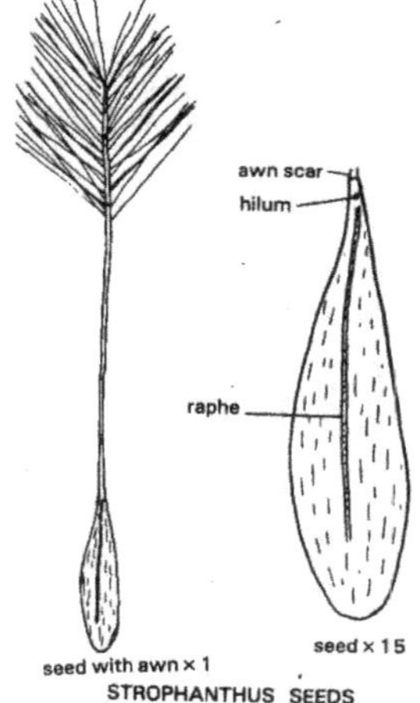

STROPHANTHUS SEEDS

Morphology: Shape – lanceolate and acuminate; Size – 1.2-1.7 cm(l) and 3 – 5 mm(b); Colour – silvery grey to yellowish green and pale brown; Fracture – short; Odour – slight, characteristic; Taste – very bitter.

Active Constituents: GLYCOSIDES – Cardiac glycosides (8 – 10%) – Cardenolides –k-strophanthin, a mixture of three glycosides viz.

    – k-strophanthoside (k-strophanthidin + cymarose + β glucose + α glucose)
    – k-strophanthin β (k-strophanthidin + cymarose + β glucose)
    – cymarin (k-strophanthidin + cymarose)

In *S. gratus* only one glycoside (4 – 8%).

    Ouabain (g-strophanthin) = Ouabagenin (g-strophanthidin) + rhamnose.

Therapeutical Uses: 1. In acute cardiac failure – In action it resembles that of *Digitails* and *Urginea* (Scilla) Glycosides, but with *Strophanthus* the action is quick and intensive. 2. Increases blood pressure. 3. Diuretic (stimulates the flow of urine) in cardiac edema.

Adulterant: Recent market samples of Strophanthus invariably consisted of seeds of *Holarrhena antidysenterica* (Kurchi seeds) (Fam. Apocynaceae). These however, can be distinguished from authentic drug on the basis of their external –, internal characters and TLC studies. Externally Kurchi seeds are dark brown and glabrous; in T.S. they show highly convoluted cotyledons; presence of conessine and other alkaloids can easily be confirmed by chemical tests and TLC studies.

TAMARIND

Source: Tamarind consists of dried ripe fruits of *Tamarindus indica* L. freed from the brittle epicarp (Fam. Leguminosae).

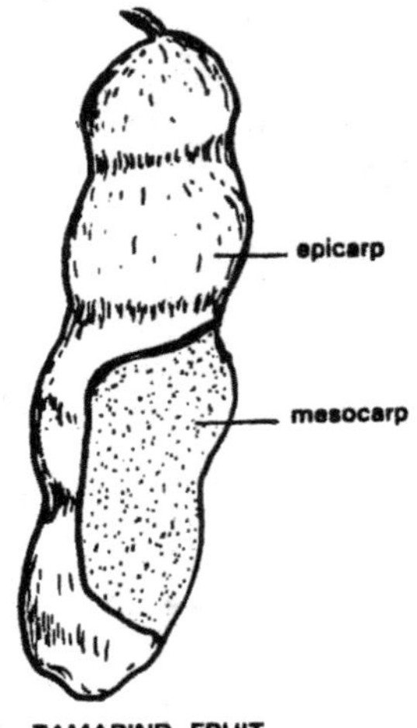

TAMARIND FRUIT

Synonyms and Regional Names: Ben. Tentul, Guj Amli, Hin. Imli. Amli, Kan. Hunise hannu, Mal. Amlam Puli, Mar. Ambli, Chinch, San. Amlika, Tam. Puliyam, Tel. Chinta pandu.

Morphology: Form – moist, sour cum sugary mass embedding fibrous strands and large reddish brown, hard, non-endospermous, glossy seeds. Odour – characteristic and Taste – pleasantly acidic and sweet.

Active Constituents: Organic acids (10%) and their salts – Tartaric acid – Citric acid – Maleic acid – Sodium and Potassium tartarate (8%), Invert sugars (30 – 40%).

Therapeutical Uses: 1. Mild laxative   2. In confection of Senna.

TANNIC ACID

Source: Tannic acid is obtained from Nutgalls which in turn are vegetable growths found on the young twigs of *Quercus infectoria* (Fam. Fagaceae). These vegetable growths are formed as a result of the deposition of the eggs of Gall-wasp (*Adleria gallae-tinctoriae*). The galls are to be powdered and then extracted with ether: alcohol (4:1) mixture; and to which water is added later. The liquid now separates into two layers. The aqueous layer contains gallo-tannin (tannic acid) and the ether layer free gallic acid. On evaporation of the solution of gallotannin, the tannic acid is purified.

Nature: Amorphous powder, yellow white to brown in colour with feeble odour and strongly astringent taste. Solubility – soluble in water, acetone, alcohol but insoluble in ether and chloroform.

Chemical Nature: Gallic acid is the mixture of esters of glucose with gallic acid. This hydrolysable tannin eventually yields on hydrolysis gallic acid and glucose.

Therapeutical and Pharmaceutical Uses: 1. Being an astringent, it is used externally in the treatment of burns.   2. In cases of alkaloidal poisoning.

TAR

Source: Tar is obtained by destructive distillation of the wood of different species of *Pinus.* (Fam. Pinaceae). Tar IP is a bituminous liquid obtained from the wood of various trees of the family Pinaceae, chiefly *Pinus longifolia,* by destructive distillation.

Synonyms: Pine tar, Pix liquida, Stockholm tar, Wood tar.

Nature: Black or dark brown semi liquid with characteristic or naphthalene like odour and with acrid and pungent taste. Some attribute the burned smell of an animal or plant as a peculiarity of its odour. Insoluble in water, partly soluble in alcohol, more soluble in chloroform, ether, fixed oils and volatile oils.

Active Constituents: MIXTURE OF PHENOLS – phenol, cresol, methyl cresol, catechol, guaiacol etc.
HYDROCARBONS – benzene, toluene, xylene, styrene, naphthalene etc.

Therapeutical and Pharmaceutical Uses: Applied externally on skin as: 1. Sedative antiseptic   2. Antibacterial   3. Local irritant and   4. Also as an expectorant in higher doses.

Chemical Tests: Litmus test. 1 g of tar is taken in 20 ml of water and shaken for some time. Filter and the filtrate is acidic to litmus.

To 5 ml of the above filtrate add 0.1% of ferric chloride and observe red colouration.

TRAGACANTH

Source: Tragacanth is the dried gummy exudation obtained from the stem of *Astragalus gummifer* Labill. (Fam. Leguminosae).

Synonyms and Regional Names: Gum Tragacanth, Hin. Anjira.

Morphology: Form – flattened, lamellated, tough ribbon shaped pieces of horny structures, more or less curved or contorted; Colour – white or faint yellow; Size – about 2.5 cm(l); Fracture – short; Odour – none; Taste – insipid and mucilaginous.

Active Constituents: CARBOHYDRATE – a complex polysaccharide
– water soluble Tragacanthin (30 to 40%)
– water insoluble Bassorin (60 to 70%)
   Tragacanthin in turn consists of (a) tragacanthic acid + (galacturonic acid + xylose + fucose + galactose) and (b) Arabinogalactan + (arabinose + galactose + galacturonic acid + rhamnose in small quantities)
Tragacanth also contains 3% starch and cellulose.

Therapeutical and Pharmaceutical Uses: 1. Used as a demulcent (soothing) 2. Suspending agent   3. Binding agent   4. Emulsifying agent   5. Laxative.

Chemical Tests

1. Solubility – Partially soluble in water (distinction from Acacia & Agar).
2. On warming Tragacanth in a soln. of alcoholic potash a canary yellow colour is obtained. (distinction from Sterculia).
3. Greenish colour is obtained after boiling Tragacanth with strong iodine soln.
4. On mounting a small amount of the powdered drug in ruthenium red, it is not stained (Distinction from Agar and Sterculia).
5. Test for reducing sugars; To 4 ml of the aqueous soln. of Tragacanth, 1 ml of dil. HCl is added and heated on a water bath for 30 minutes. Divide this into two portions. To one portion of the resulting hydrolyzed mixture, 1.5 ml of NaOH is added to neutralize and again reheated with 3 ml of Fehling's solution whereby a red ppt. is formed indicating the presence of sugars. To the other portion a few ml of barium chloride soln. is added whereby no ppt. is formed (distinction from Agar).
6. On boiling 1 g with 20 ml of water, a mucilage is formed. Addition of a few drops of fresh lead acetate soln. to 1 ml of this mucliage, white ppt. is seen (distinction from Acacia).

Substitutes and Adulterants: 1. Sterculia gum also called, Indian Tragacanth or Karaya gum is a substitute and official in some Pharmacopoeias. It is a dried gummy exudation obtained from the stem of *Sterculia urens* (Fam. Sterculiaceae). It is pathological in origin and used as a bulk laxative. In some properties it resembles Tragacanth and therefore erroneously called Indian Tragacanth. The gum occurs in irregular translucent, striated, occasionally vermiform pieces, white to brown to purple in colour; at times small fragments of bark may be attached. It has acetic acid odour. With water it forms colourless, transparent jelly. Some important differences between tragacanth and sterculia are tabulated below:

2. *Katira gum:* This appears in commerce as karaya gum. It is derived from *Cochlospermum gossypium* (Fam. Cochlospermaceae). The gum contains calcium oxalate crystal on the basis of which it is possible to distinguish this from others.

Parameters	Tragacanth *Astragalus gummifer* (Leguminosae)	Sterculia *Sterculia urens* (Sterculiaceae)
Odour	not characteristic	marked acetic acid odour
Iodine test	starch present	absent
Ruthenium Red	no action	stains pink, mucilage present
Solubility in water	swells to gelatinous mass and becomes adhesive	low solubility but swells to many times to original volume becomes quite brittle
When boiled with solution of potash	canary yellow colour	slightly brownish colour
When hydrolysed with 5% phosphoric acid, has the volatile acidity	2 – 3%	not less than 14%
Methoxy value	30 – 40	zero

TULSI

Source: Tulsi is the fresh and dried leaves of *Ocimum* species like *O. sanctum* L., *O. basilicum* L. etc. (Fam. Labiatae).

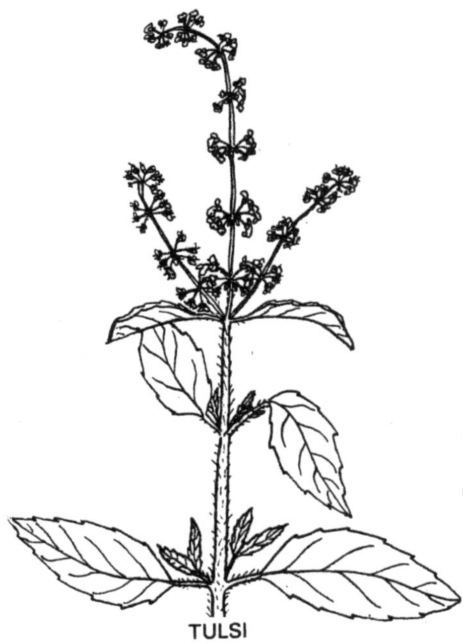

Synonyms and Regional Names: Sacred basil, Tulsi, Kali-tulsi, Varanda.

Morphology: Leaves (Green type of *O. sanctum*): Exstipulate, opposite, petiolate. Petiole 2.5 to 3.0 cm(l), slender, thin, pubescent with narrow adaxial groove; lamina elliptical to ovoid, oblong 5 – 6 cm(l) and 2.5 to 3 cm(b), pubescent; margin entire, irregularly undulated or bluntly serrate; apex acute or obtuse; adaxial surface bright green; abaxial surface pale green with prominent veins, venation pinnately reticulate with 5 – 6 alternate pairs of lateral veins; glandular dots seen minutely on the abaxial side; Odour – aromatic and Taste – pungent.

Leaves (Purple type of *O. sanctum*): Opposite, exstipulate, petiolate. Petiole green with purplish tinge, 3.5 cm(l); slender, thin, less pubescent with narrow inconspicuous adaxial groove; lamina elliptic to oblong, 5 – 7 cm(l), 2.5 to 3.5 cm(b), margin narrowly or distantly serrate, apex acute or obtuse, almost glabrous except at veins, aromatic with pungent taste, venation pinnately reticulate with 5 – 7 lateral alternate pairs of veins, adaxial side dark green, abaxial side dull green, veins prominent on both surfaces; Odour – aromatic and Taste – pungent.

Active Constituents: ESSENTIAL OIL (0.7%) – phenols (eugenol 70%), nerol, eugenol methyl ether, caryophyllene, terpinene-4-Ol – decylaldehyde, r-selinene, α-& β pinene – camphor and carvacrol.

Therapeutical and Pharmaceutical Uses: 1. Expectorant – in cases of catarrh and bronchitis 2. Stomachic, carminative, refrigerent and febrifuge 3. Antibacterial, insecticidal and antiprotozoal 4. Antifertility agent.

TURMERIC

Sources: Turmeric consists of the dried rhizomes of *Curcuma longa* L. (Fam. Zingiberaceae).

Synonyms and Regional Names: Curcuma, Indian Saffron, Ben. Halud, Guj. Halada, Hin. Haldi, Kan. Arisina, San. Haldi, Haridra, Tam. Manjal, Tel. Pasupu.

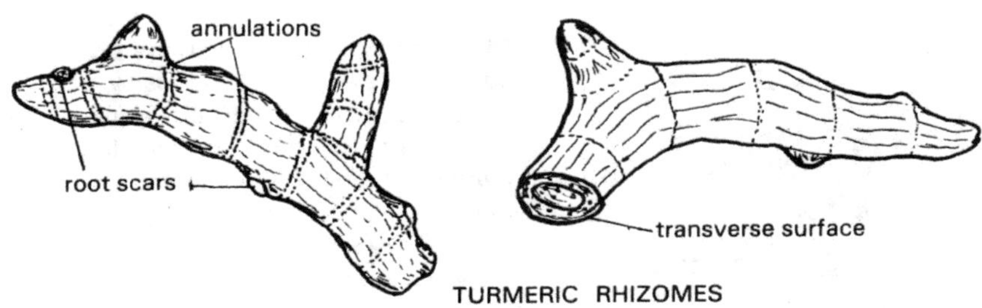

TURMERIC RHIZOMES

Morphology. Form – primary rhizomes ovate, oblong or pyriform and are called in commerce as 'bulb' or 'round turmeric'; whereas the lateral rhizomes are more cylindrical and often short, branched and they are called 'long turmeric'. Colour – yellow to yellowish brown externally, yellow to yellow orange internally. Size – the round form is about half as broad as 'long'. The long forms are about 4 to 7 cm(l) and 1 to 1.5 cm(w); Surface – root scars and annulations are seen, Fracture – horny; Odour – aromatic; Taste – aromatic and bitter.

Active Constituents: CURCUMINOIDS (non-volatile colouring matter – 5%)
– curcumin, a diferuloylmethane – desmethoxy curcumin, a dicinnamoylmethane
– bidesmethoxy curcumin
VOLATILE OIL (5%) – sesquiterpenes (60%) like-1-cycloisoprenmyrcene
   – zingiberene (25)%, tumerone, ar-tumerone, α atlantone, γ atlantone
   – phellandrene, sabinene, and so also cineole, borneol and curcumone
SUGARS – arabinose (1%), fructose (12%) and glucose (28%)
Bitter substances, fixed oil and acids.

Therapeutical and Pharmaceutical Uses: 1. Choleretic and cholagogue 2. Anti-inflammatory agent 3. Aromatic, stimulant, tonic and carminative 4. Anti-fertility agent 5. In respiratory diseases 6. To lower the blood cholesterol level 7. Externally applied in pains and bruises 8. As a colouring agent 9. In cosmetics 10. Anti-microbial.

Chemical Tests (as per IPC): 1. Con. H_2SO_4 or a mixture of H_2SO_4 with alcohol (90%) imparts a deep crimson colour to turmeric 2. Boric acid colours to reddish brown which on addition of alkalies becomes greenish blue.

TURPENTINE OIL

Source. Turpentine oil is the volatile oil distilled from the oleo-resin obtained from *Pinus palustris* Miller and from other species of *Pinus* (Fam. Pinaceae) which yield terpene oils exclusively.

Nature: Colour – colourless, limpid liquid; Odour – strong and characteristic; Taste – pungent, somewhat bitter. On exposure to air and on storage, odour and taste become strong and less pleasant.

Active Constituents: VOLATILE OIL (13 to 30%) – α pinene (64%) – β pinene (33%) and in traces dipentene, methylchavicol, bornyl acetate.

Therapeutical and Pharmaceutical Uses: 1. Mild antiseptic 2. Counter irritant 3. Insecticide 4. Expectorant in bronchitis 5. In the Preparation of synthetic camphor.

INDIAN SQUILL (URGINEA)

Source: Urginea is the bulb of *Urginea indica* Kunth, *(Drimia indica)* Fam. Liliaceae, divested of its dry membranous outer scales, cut into slices and dried.

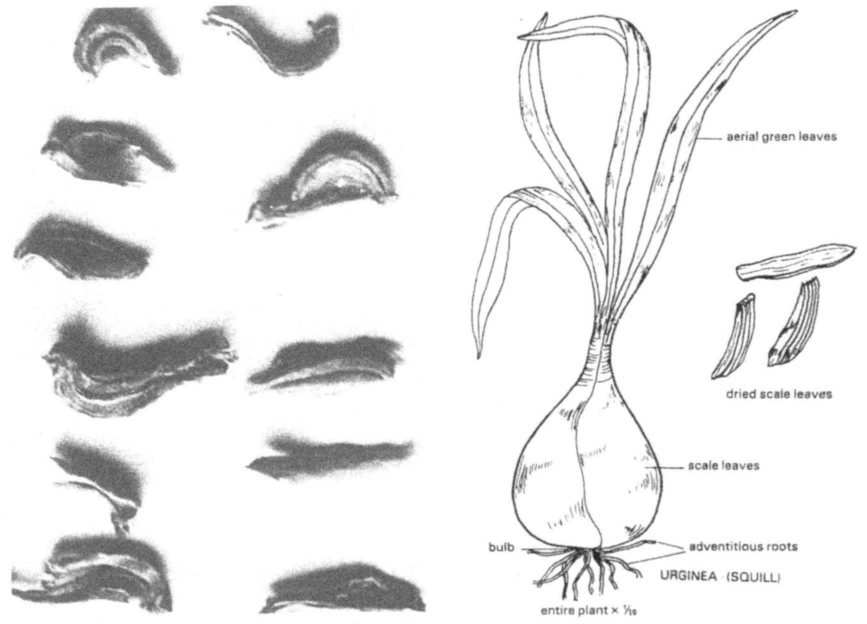

Urginea – scale leaves

Synonyms and Regional Names: Indian Squill, Ben. Guj. Hin. Jangli piyaz; Kan. Kadu bellulli; Mal. Kantena; Mar. Bhuikanda; San. Vanapalandam, Kolakanda; Tam. Narivengayam; Tel. Adavi-tellagadd.

Morphology: Form – curved or irregularly shaped strips frequently tapering towards the ends; occasionally grouped, 3 to 4 together and attached to a portion of the axis; Colour – pale yellowish brown to buff; Size – 1 – 5 cm(l), 3 – 10 mm(w) and 1 – 3 mm(t); Surface ridged longitudinally; Fracture – brittle when dry, but tough and flexible when damp; Odourless and Taste—mucilaginous and bitter.

Active Constituents

GLYCOSIDES   – Cardiac glycosides, Burfadienolides (Scilladienolides)

WHITE RACE   – Glucoscillaren A ⎤   AGLYCONES
– Scillaren A   ⎬   Scillarenin
– Proscillaridin A ⎦

– Scilliroside   →⎤   Scillirosidin
RED RACE   – Scillirubroside →⎦   Scillirubrosidin

Therapeutical and Pharmaceutical Uses: 1. In heart ailments – oldage, insufficiency of aorta. 2. Diuretic (stimulates the flow of urine) in cardiac edema. 3. Rodenticide (rat poison) exhibited by the active constituent (Scilliroside) of red race only.

VAJ

Source: Vaj consists of the dried peeled and unpeeled rhizomes of *Acorus calamus* L. (Fam. Araceae).

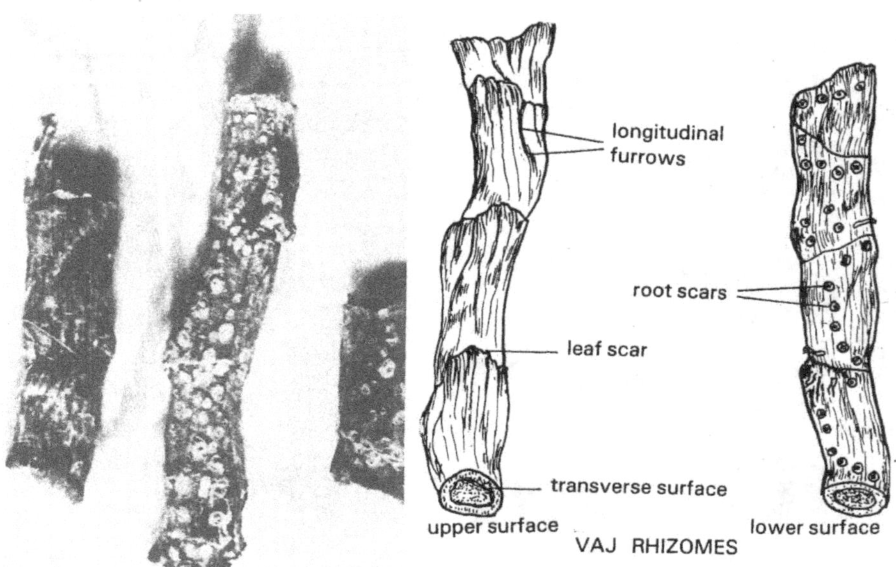

VAJ RHIZOMES

Synonyms and Regional Names: Calamus root, Sweet flag, Ben. Hin. Bach; Guj. Godavaj; Kan. Baje; Mal. Vayambhu; Mar. Vekhand; Tam. Vasambu; Tel. Vasa.

Morphology: Form – subcylindrical, split longitudinally; Colour – pale yellowish to pinkish brown; Size – upto 22 cm(l), 2 cm(t); Surface – longitudinally furrowed (upper), dark coloured slightly raised root scars in zigzag arrangement (lower); Fracture – short, granular and porous; Odour – aromatic; Taste – aromatic, bitter, acrid.

Active Constituents: VOLATILE OIL (1.5 – 3.5%) – α-asarone and β-asarone (8 – 19%). These are trans and cis isomers respectively of 2-4-5-trimethoxy-1-propanyl-benzene.

Shyobunone – like Sesquiterpenoids (4 to 8%).

Therapeutical and Pharmaceutical Uses: 1. Stomachic, antispasmodic and carminative 2. Sedative (tranquillizer) 3. Antifungal, antibacterial and insecticidal 4. Significant relief in bronchospasm 5. Vaj is used in 51 drug preparations (Kapoor & Mitra).

VALERIAN (INDIAN)

Source: Indian Valerian consists of the dried rhizomes, stolons and roots of *Valeriana wallichii* DC. (Fam. Valerianaceae).

Synonyms and Regional Names: Ben. Tagar; Hin. Tagar; Kan. Mandibattal; Mar. Tagar-ganthoda; San. Tagar.

Morphology: Rhizomes; Colour – yellowish brown; Form – subcylindrical, dorsiventrally flattened, slightly curved and unbranched; Uppersurface – prominent leaf scars and undersurface – circular root scars with a few thick roots; Fracture – short and horny; Odour – very characteristic; Taste – bitter.

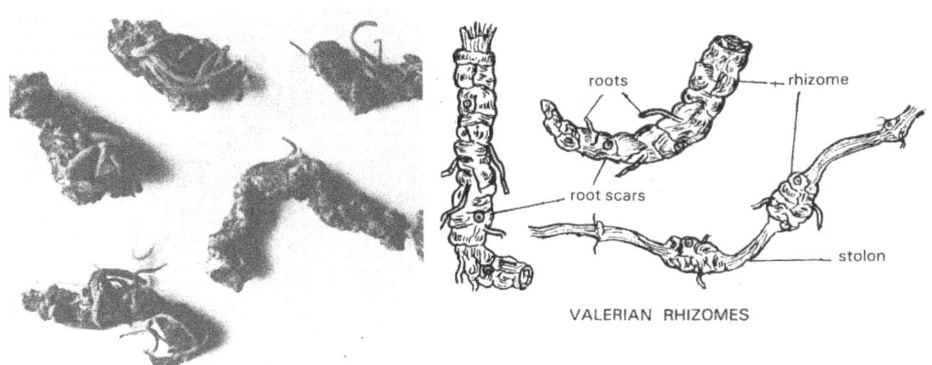

VALERIAN RHIZOMES

Active Constituents: VALEPOTRIATES (0.5 – 3%) Cyclopenta (c) – pyran with an epoxy triester structure – Valtratum – Didrovaltratum – Acevaltratum – Isovaleroxy – hydroxy – didrovaltratum
ESSENTIAL OIL (0.5 – 1.5%)
VALERIOSIDAT, a water soluble iridoid ester glycoside without epoxide ring
ALKALOIDS in traces (not active).

Therapeutical and Pharmaceutical Uses: 1. Sedative (calms down activity and excitement) 2. Depressent effect on CNS 3. Remedy for Hysteria, Hypochondriasis (unnecessary anxiety about one's own health with pessimistic imaginations) and nervous unrest.

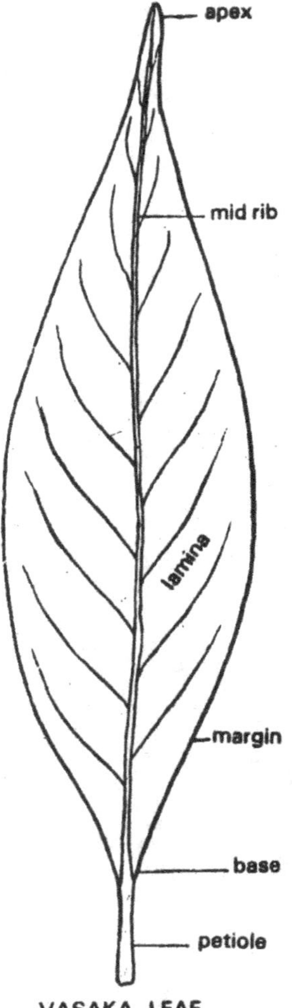

VASAKA LEAF

VASAKA

Source: Vasaka consists of the fresh and dried leaves of *Adhatoda vasica* Nees. (Fam. Acanthaceae).

Synonyms and Regional Names
Ben.　Bakas
Guj.　Adsoge
Hin.　Arusha
Kan.　Adusoge
Mal.　Adalodagam
Mar.　Adulsa
San.　Vasika, Vasa,
　　　Sinmukhi
Tam.　Adatodai
Tel.　Addasaramu

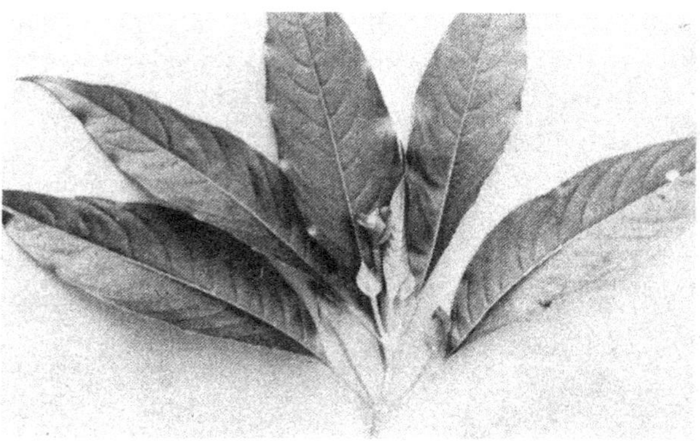

Morphology: Type-simple; Colour – dark green; Shape – lanceolate; Size – 12-20 cm(l) 2.5 – 5 cm(b); Petiole – petiolate, margin entire, apex acuminate, base acute and equal, venation reticulate; Upper surface glabrous and lower surface pale green and glabrous; Odour – characteristic and Taste – bitter.

Active Constituents: ALKALOIDS (0.25%) – Quinazoline type – Vasicine (Peganine) – Oxyvasicine (6-oxypeganine) – Vasicinone – Ketone (oxidation product of vasicine)
ESSENTIAL OIL
— Adhatodic acid, Vasakin, an insecticide of unknown nature, etc. According to Atal et. al(1980) the activity of the drug lies only in Vasicine and Vasicinone.

Therapeutical and Pharmaceutical Uses: 1. Expectorant   2. Bronchodilator 3. Oxytocic   4. As an abortifacient   5. Vasaka is used 110 drug preparations (Kapoor & Mitra).

VIDANG

Source: Vidang consists of the dried fruits of *Embelia ribes* Burn. (Fam. Myrsinaceae).

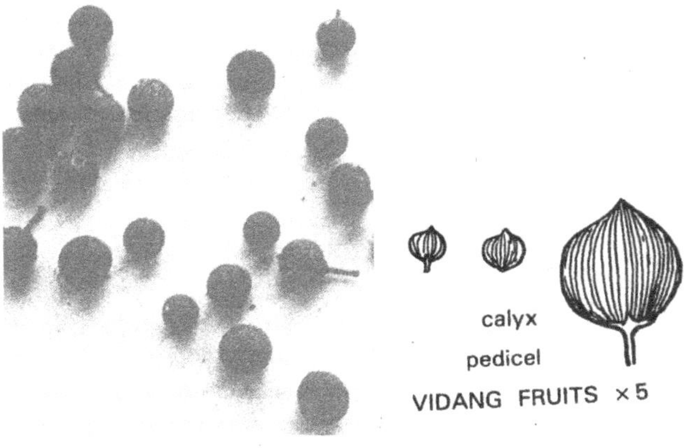

Synonyms and Regional Names
Embelia
Ben. Biranga
Guj. Hin. Karkannie
Kan. Vayuvilanga
Mar. Vavadinga
San. Bidanga
Tam. Vaayuvilangam
Tel. Vellal

Morphology
Form – spherical or globular; Colour – varies from red to nearly black; Size – 4 mm(d); Surface – warty, a short pedicel and a small 5-partite calyx may or may not be present, when absent they are represented by small holes. Brittle pericarp encloses a red seed. Odour and Taste – faintly aromatic and astringent.

Active Constituents: QUINONE – Embelin (2.5%) (embelic acid) – Vilangin.

Therapeutical and Pharmaceutical Uses: 1. Anthelmintic against tape worm. 2. Antifertility agent.

Chemical Test: Shake 0.2 g of vidang powder in 5 ml ether, filter and to the filtrate on adding one to two drops of dil. ammonia, a bluish violet ppt. is seen.

Substitutes and Adulterants: Market samples of Vidang contain invariably a very high proportion of one another species namely, *E. robusta (syn. E. tsjeriam-cottam)* also called red vidang. This species also contains the active principles as much as 1.6% besides a small amount of essential oil and therefore is a good substitute. These red coloured fruits are bigger, elongated tangentially and with longitudinal wrinkles. Calyx with 5 sepals is easily seen. Characteristic features are the presence of volatile oil glands in the outer mesocarp and 3 to 6 layers of stone cells in the inner mesocarp and these features are totally absent in the official species.

VINCA

Source: Vinca is the whole plant of *Catharanthus roseus* L. (Fam. Apocynaceae).

Synonyms and Regional Names: *Vinca rosea, Lochnera rosea,* Sadaphuli, Rattanjot Billaganneru.

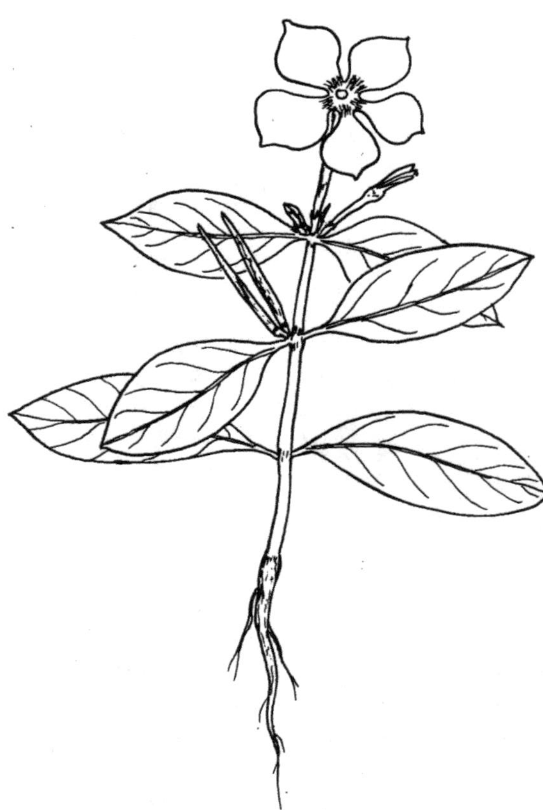

VINCA PLANT × ¼

Morphology of the entire plant: Type – Annular or perennial herb; Size – 0.5 to 1 m(l), Leaves – ovate, oblong, glossy above glaucous below; Flowers – 2 – 3 in cymes, axillary and terminal clusters. Based on the flower colour, three varieties are known namely – *alba* – white, *ocullata* – white with pink or carmine red eyes and *roseus* – with rose coloured flowers. Fruit – a follicle, cylindrical and many seeded.

Active Constituents: ALKALOIDS – (roots 0.85%, leaves 0.67%, stems 0.31%) – Indole and Indoline alkaloids – Ajmalicine, Lochnerine, Serpentine and Tetrahydroalstonine – Dimeric Indole bases of Monoterpene types – Vinblastine – Vincristine.

Therapeutical and Pharmaceutical Uses: 1. Antineoplastic (antimitotic = anticancer = cytostatic = antitumour) agents 2. In the treatment of Hodgkin's disease 3. In the treatment of leukaemia in children.

128

WILD CHERRY BARK

Source: Wild Cherry Bark is the dried bark of *Prunus serotina* Ehrhart. collected in autumn (Fam. Rosaceae).

Synonyms: Virginian bark, Virginian, Prune bark.

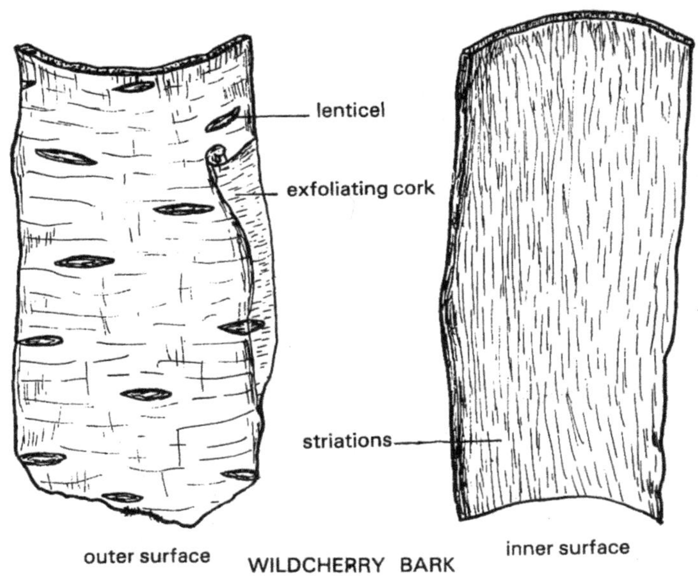

Morphology: Shape – flat, curved or channelled pieces; Colour – reddish brown to dark brown on the outer side; Size – upto 10 cm(l), 5 cm(b), upto 3 mm(t); Outer surface – covered with a smooth exfoliating papery cork containing numerous transversely elongated lenticels. Inner surface – fine, irregular longitudinal striations are seen; Fracture – short and granular; Odour – slight, stronger when soaked in water, resembling the smell of bitter almonds; Taste – astringent and bitter.

Active Constituents: GLYCOSIDE – Cyanogenetic glycoside – Prunasin
COUMARIN derivatives – Scopoletin.

Therapeutical and Pharmaceutical Use: Used as sedative in cough preparations.

Chemical Test: Moisten with water 1 g of powdered drug (even broken pieces of drug will do). This is now taken in a special test tube with a split cork. Insert a piece of sodium picrate paper into the split cork. Allow to stand for about 30 min. If HCN is present in the drug, it gives the picrate paper a brick red colour.

APPENDIX – I

(Active Constituents and the drugs containing them)

Alkaloids
Aconite
Aswagandha
Banafsha
Belladonna
Cinchona
Cocaine
Colchicum
Datura herb
Ephedra
Ergot
Gentian
Hyoscyamus
Ipecac
Kurchi
Lobelia
Nux vomica
Opium
Pipal
Physostigma
Punarnava
Rauwolfia
Shankhpushpi
Vasaka
Vinca

Anthracene Glycosides
Aloes
Cascara
Chrysarobin
Rhubarb
Senna

Balsamic Acids
Balsam of Tolu
Benzoin
Storax

Bitter Principles
Chirata
Gentian
Kalmegh
Picrorhiza
Quassia

Carbohydrates
Acacia
Aga

Alginate
Cotton
Guar gum
Honey
Pectin
Starch
Tragacanth

Cardiac Glycosides
Digitalis
Strophanthus
Urginea

Cyanogenetic Glycosides
Bitter almond
Linseed
Wild cherry bark

Esters
Pyrethrum

Flavonoids (Glycosides)
Bavchi
Catechu
Lemon peel
Licorice
Orange peel
Podophyllum
Rasna

Furocoumarins
Bael
Bavchi

Glycosides General
Aloes
Cascara
Chrysarobin
Digitalis
Ipomoea
Kaladana
Licorice
Quillaia
Rhubarb
Senna
Strophanthus
Urginea
Wild cherry bark

Lipids/Fixed Oils/Fats/Wax
Arachis Oil
Bees Wax
Castor Oil
Chaulmoogra Oil
Ergot
Kokum Butter
Lanolin
Linseed
Mustard
Sesame Oil
Shark-liver Oil

Mucilage
Agar
Isapgol
Linseed

Oleo-Gum-Resin
Asafetida
Myrrh

Oleo-Resin
Male Fern

Organic Acid
Tamarind

Protein
Gelatin

Pungent Principles
Capsicum
Ginger
Pipal

Quinones
Vidang

Resins
Balsam of Tolu
Cannabis
Colocynth
Colophony
Ipomoea ⎫
Jalap   ⎬ Resinous Glycosides
Kaladana ⎭
Podophyllum
Rasna
Rhubarb

Saponin Glycosides
Banafsha
Brahmi
Dioscorea
Gokhru
Licorice
Quillaia
Satavari
Senega

Tannins
Amla
Arjuna
Asoka
Bael
Bahera
Catechu (black & pale)
Myrobalan
Rasna
Tannic acid

Terpenoids
Artemisia
Camphor

Volatile Oils
Artemisia
Bavchi
Bitter almond Oil
Caraway
Cardamom
Cassia
Chenopodium Oil
Cinnamon
Clove
Coriander
Dill
Eucalyptus
Fennel
Ginger
Jatamansi

Kapur Kachri
Kesar
Lehsun
Lemongrass Oil
Lemon peel
Mentha Oil
Mustard Oil
Nutmeg
Orange peel
Pipal
Pudina
Rasna
Tulsi
Turmeric
Turpentine Oil
Vaj
Valerian
Vasaka

APPENDIX – II

(List of drugs classified according to their therapeutic activity)

Abortifacient
Nutmeg
Vasaka

Analgesic
Aconite
Bavchi (Bavachinine)
Cannabis
Opium

Anthelmintic
Artemisia
Bavchi
Chenopodium Oil
Kalmegh
Kapur Kachri
Male Fern
Quassia

Antiasthmatic
Ephedra
Lobelia
Saussurea
Shankhpushpi
Vasaka

Antiatherosclerotic
Lehsun

Antibacterial
Amla
Aswagandha
Bavchi (essential oil)
Brahmi
Cannabis
Eucalyptus
Lehsun
Rasna

Antidiarrhoetic
Bael
Isapgol
Kurchi
Pale Catechu
Pectin
Rhubarb

Antidysenteric
Ipecac
Isapgol
Kalmegh

Kurchi
Shankhpushpi

Antifungal
Amla
Bavchi (essential oil)
Pudina
Rasna

Antihypertensive
Lehsun
Rauwolfia

Antileprotic
Chaulmoogra oil

Antiinflammatory
Bavchi
Colchicum
Kapur Kachri
Licorice
Punarnava

Antimalarial
Cinchona

Antimenorrhegia
Asoka

Antimigraine
Ergot

Antimuscarinic
Belladonna
Datura
Hyoscyamus

Antiperiodic
Kurchi
Picrorhiza

Antipruritic
Camphor
Capsicum

Antirheumatic
Aconite
Rasna

Antiseptic
Balsam of Tolu
Benzoin
Camphor
Chrysarobin
Clove
Myrrh
Pudina
Turpentine Oil

Antisialagogue
Belladonna
Datura
Hyoscyamus

Antispasmodic
Amla
Asafetida
Belladonna
Caraway
Datura
Fennel
Hyoscyamus
Kapur Kachri
Kesar
Licorice
Mentha oil

Antituberculotic
Chaulmoogra oil
Eucalyptus

Antitumors
Aswagandha
Lehsun
Podophyllum
Vinca

Aphrodisiac
Asafetida
Aswagandha
Cinnamon
Gokhru
Kapur Kachri
Nux vomica

Astringent
Amla
Arjuna
Asoka
Bahera
Catechu
Kokum butter
Tannic acid

Bitter Tonic
Chirata
Gentian
Kalmegh
Picrorhiza
Orange peel
Quassia
Shankhpushpi

Cardiotonic
Digitalis
Strophanthus
Urginea

Carminative
Asafetida
Camphor
Capsicum
Caraway
Cardamom
Coriander
Dill
Fennel
Ginger
Lehsun
Mentha Oil
Nutmeg
Pipal

Pudina
Rasna

Cathartic
Aloes
Cascara
Castor oil
Podophyllum
(only American)
Rhubarb
Senna

Cholagogue
Picrorhiza
Mentha oil

Demulcent
Acacia
Honey
Isapgol
Licorice
Linseed
Sesame oil
Starch
Tragacanth

Diaphoretic
Banafsha
Eucalyptus

Digestant
Gentian
Lehsun

Diuretic
Amla
Arjuna
Banafsha
Gokhru
Punarnava

Emetic
Ipecac

Emmenagogue
Kapur Kachri
Kesar

Emollient
Arachis Oil
Lanolin
Kokum Butter
Linseed Oil
Sesame Oil

Expectorant
Asafetida
Balsam of Tolu
Banafsha
Benzoin
Eucalyptus
Ipecac
Licorice
Pudina
Senega
Turpentine Oil
Vasaka

Febrifuge
Arjuna
Chirata
Kalmegh
Picrorhiza

Flavouring Agent
Bitter almond
Cassia
Cardamom
Cinnamom
Clove
Coriander
Ginger
Kesar
Lehsun
Lemon peel
Lémongrass oil
Nutmeg
Orange peel
Pudina
Saussurea

Galactagogue
Fennel
Satavari

Germicide
Cassia (oil)
Cinnamon (oli)

Hypnotic
Cannabis
Opium

Insecticide
Pyrethrum
Quassia
Turpentine oil

Laxative
Agar
Aloes
Cascara
Guar gum
Isapgol
Myrobalan
Picrorhiza
Rhubarb
Senna

Local Anaesthetic
Cocaine

Mydriatic
Belladonna
Datura
Hyoscyamus

Nervines
Aswagandha
Belladonna
Cannabis
Capsicum
Nux vomica
Rauwolfia

Nutritive
Honey
Kokum Butter
Starch

Oxytocic
Ergot
Vasaka

Pharmaceutical Aid
Acacia
Alginate
Agar
Arachis oil
Bees wax
Colophony
Cotton
Gelatin
Guar gum
Honey
Kaolin
Kokum Butter
Lanolin
Lemon peel
Lemongrass oil
Orange peel

Starch
Storax

Protective
Guar gum
Linseed
Starch

Psychotropic
Cannabis
Opium

Rubefacient
Mustard oil

Sedative
Aswagandha
Belladonna
Brahmi
Camphor
Cannabis
Datura
Fennel
Hyoscyamus
Jatamansi
Kesar
Myrrh
Rauwolfia
Valerian
Wild cherry bark
(cough-)

Stimulant
Aswagandha
Clove
Cocaine
Coriander
Dill
Ginger
Kesar
Myrrh
Nux vomica
Pipal
Rasna
Rauwolfia
Storax

Stomachic
Chirata
Kalmegh
Kapur Kachri
Kesar

Lehsun
Nux vomica
Picrorhiza
Pipal
Rasna

Tonic
Amla (liver tonic)

Vehicle for Oily Injections
Arachis Oil

Bitter almond oil
Sesame Oil

Vesicant
Cantharides

INDEX TO PLANT (animal) GENERA AND SPECIES

135

BIBLIOGRAPHY

Pharmacopoeia of India: Government of India Publication (1966).

Indian Pharmaceutical Codex: B. Mukerji, C.S.I.R. Publication, 1 (1953).

Lehrbuch der Pharmakognosie: E. Stahl, Gustav Fischer Verlag, Stuttgart (1962).

Chromatographische und Mikroskopische Analyse von Drogen: E. Stahl, Gustav Fischer Verlag, Stuttgart (1970).

Teeanalyse: L. Hoerhammer, Springer Verlag, Berlin (1970).

Hagers Handbuch Der Pharmazeutischen Praxis: P. H. List and L. Hoerhammer Springer Verlag Berlin – Heidelberg (1971), Vol. 1, 2, 3, 4 (1971 – 74).

Text Book of Pharmacognosy: T. E. Wallis, J. & A. Churchill Ltd. London 104 Gloucester Place, W. 1 (1955).

Lehrbuch der Pharmakognosie: E. Steinegger and R. Haensel, Springer Verlag Berlin Heidelber (1972).

Modern Pharmacognosy: E, Ramstad, Mc Graw – Hill Book Company, USA (1959).

Pharmacognosy; E. P. Claus, V. E. Tyler, L. R. Brady, Lea & Febiger (Henry Kimpton, London) 7th Edn. (1976).

The Hindu Pharmacopoeia; A. R. S. Sundaram. Yogasrama, Royapettah, Madras (1933).

Chopra's Indigenous Drugs of India: R. N. Chopra, I. C. Chopra, K. L. Handa and L. D. Kapur, U. N. Dhar & Sons Private Limited, Calcutta – 12 (1958).

Pharmacognosy: G. E. Trease and W. C. Evans; Bailliere Tindall, London 11th Edn. (1978, 12th Edn. 1983).

Medicinal Plants of India and Pakistan: J. F. Dastur, D. B. Taraporevala Sons & Co. Private Ltd., Bombay (1962).

Plant Modifications: B. N. Narayana Rao, Wisdom Publications, Mysore (1972).

Pharmacognosy of Indian Root and Rhizome Drugs; S. C. Datta & B. Mukerji, Ministry of Health, Government of India's Pharmacognosy Laboratory, Calcutta (1950).

Pharmacognosy of Indian Leaf Drugs: S. C. Datta and B. Mukerji, Ministry of Health, Government of India's Pharmacognosy Laboratory, Calcutta (1952).

A Text Book of Pharmacognosy: C. S. Shah, and J. S. Quadry; Messrs B. S. Shah, Ahmedabad (1975 – 76).

Five Hundred Indian Plants: B. J. Ponon; Basel Mission Book & Tract Depository (1918)

Dr. K. M. Nadkarni's Indian Materia Medica: A. K. Nadkarni; Popular Book Depot, Bombay (1954).

Natural Products: R. Ikan, Israel Univeristy Press, Jerusalem (1969).

Chemical Plant Taxonomy: Edited by T. Swain; Academic Press; London and New York (1963).

Dorland's Pocket Medical Dictionary, Oxford & IBM Publishing Co., Calcutta (1972).

R. Schaette, Ph. D. Dissertation, Munich University, Munich (1971).

Current Research on Medicinal and Aromatic Plants: R. S. Thakur and A.Goswami 1(1), 36. (1979).

Herbal Drugs in Indian Pharmaceutical Industry: S. L. Kapoor & K. Mitra, a NBRI Lucknow Publication (1979).

Medicinal Plants of India Vo. I: ICMR Publication (1976), Vol. 2 (1987).

Anatomy of Crude Drugs: M. A. Iyengar & S. G. K. Nayak. (1975, 1979, 1984, 1987, 1991).

Single Drugs of India: N. S. Mooss, Vaidyasarathi Press Limited, Kottayam (1976)

Medicinal Plants: S. K. Jain, N. B. T. Inida (1968).

Spices and Condiments: J. S. Pruthi, N. B. T. India (1976).

Sacred Trees Across Cultures and Nations: S. S. Gupta, Indian Publication, Calcutta (1980).

Cultivation and Utilisation of Medicinal and Aromatic Plants: C. K. Atal and B. M. Kapur, RRL, Jammu – Tawi (1977).

Chemistry and Pharmacology of Vasicine – A New Oxytocic & Abortifacient: C. K. Atal, RRL, Jammu (1980).

PLANTA MEDICA issues between 1978 – 84

Medicinal & Aromatic Plants Abstracts issues 1979 – 90. Publication & Information Directorate, CSIR, New Delhi.

Bulletin of Indian Materials & Their Utilization, Publication & Information Directorate CSIR, New Delhi (1977).

Diosgenin and other Steroid Drug Precursors: L. V. Asolkar and Y. R. Chadha, Publications & Information Directorate, New Delhi (1979).

Drogen und Ihre Inhaltstoffe: H. Wagner, Gustav Fischer Verlag, Stuttgart, 1980.

An Introduction to Phytochemistry: M. S. F. Ross and K. R. Brain. Pitman Medical 1977.

Medical Botany: W. H. Lewis & M. P. F. Elvin – Lewis, John Wiley & Sons, New York (1977).

Pharmazeutische Biologie, drogenanalyse I; Morphology und Anatomie: F. Deutschmann, B. Hohmann, E. Sprecher, Egon Stahl, Gustav Fischer Verlag, Stuttgart, 1979.

Lexikon der Heilpflanzen, L. Thurzova, Lingen Verlag Köln, West Germany (1976).

Rauschgift-Drogen, H. Wagner, Springer-Verlag, Heidelberg, New York (1970).

www.ingramcontent.com/pod-product-compliance
Lightning Source LLC
LaVergne TN
LVHW021251210726
843527LV00004B/251